Practical Aspects in Veterinary Extension and Animal Husbandry

NIPA® GENX ELECTRONIC RESOURCES & SOLUTIONS P. LTD.
New Delhi-110 034

About the Authors

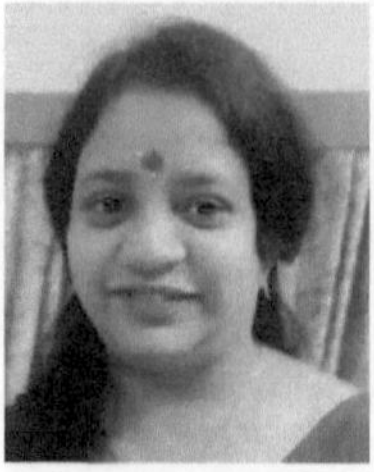

Dr. Ruchi Singh is an Assistant Professor, Department of Veterinary and Animal Husbandry Extension, College of Veterinary Science and Animal Husbandry, Nanaji Deshmukh Veterinary Science University, Jabalpur, Madhya Pradesh, India. Basically a Veterinary Extension graduate, she did her PhD, from NDRI, Karnal, Haryana and M.V.Sc. in Veterinary Extension Education from Lala Lajpat Rai University of Veterinary and Animal Science, Hisar, Haryana. She was awarded JRF by UGC.

Dr. R.Singh has worked in various capacities as Farm Manager, in Central Poultry Development Organization (ER), Bhubaneswar, Orissa, Govt. of India, Ministry of Agriculture. She taught Veterinary Extension at the undergraduate and postgraduate levels, and also conducted various extension programme of the university in rural areas of Madhya Pradesh.

Dr. Singh published more than 28 research papers in national and international journal. Dr. Singh has authored two book, one in English language named 'Content Analysis of Animal Husbandry News' and one in Hindi languages named as 'Prasar Shiksha'.

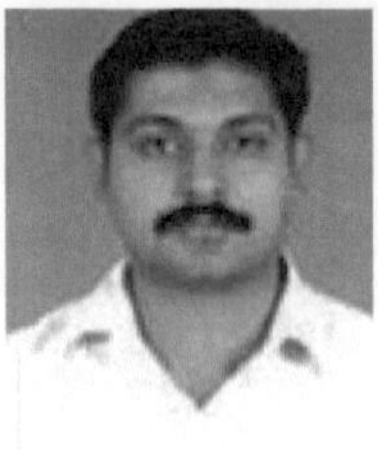

Dr. Hari R., is an assistant professor currently employed with the College of Veterinary Science and A.H., Jabalpur, in the Department of Veterinary and Animal Husbandry Extension Education. He received his Bachelor of Veterinary Science and Animal Health degree and his Master of Veterinary Science degrees from the College of Veterinary and Animal Sciences, Mannuthy in Thrissur, Kerala. He received his PhD from Indian Veterinary Research Institute, Izzatnagar in Bareilly. He was awarded the UGC-JRF and the ICAR SRF during his academic life in order to pursue his doctoral degree. He has more than eight years experience in the academic sector after his doctoral degree. He had corporate experience in addition to academic sector experience, working for a pet insurance company with a UK base. In addition to teaching, he has written 26 research articles and numerous extension articles.

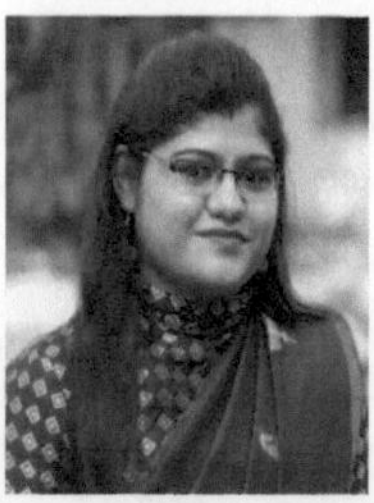

Dr. Rashmi Vishwakarma has completed her B.V.Sc & amp; A.H in 2015, M.V.Sc in 2017 and currently pursuing her PhD in Veterinary & amp; Animal Husbandry Extension from College of Veterinary Science & amp; Animal Husbandry, Jabalpur (M.P). She worked as Teaching Associate in Veterinary Polytechnic, N.D.V.S.U, Jabalpur from 2018 to 2021, she has also involved in various extension activities. She has published more than 10 research papers in national and international journals along with that more than 34 extension literatures including popular articles, training manuals, practical manuals, booklets. She is the author of a book "Pashuchikitsa Aushadhi Vigyan" published in hindi.

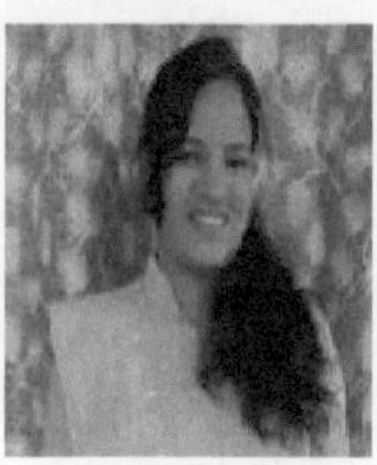

Dr. Manju Sahu has completed her B.V.Sc. and A.H. in 2016 from Chhattisgarh Kamdhenu Vishwavidyalaya, Anjora, Durg (CG). She has completed M.V.Sc. in 2018 from Orrisa University of Agriculture and Technology, Bhubaneswar and currently pursuing PhD in Veterinary Extension Education from Faculty of Veterinary and Animal Science, Banaras Hindu University, Varanasi (UP). She worked as Teaching Associate in College of Veterinary Science and Animal Husbandry, NDVSU, Jabalpur (MP) from 2019 to 2021 and also worked as Part Time Teacher in College of Veterinary Science and Animal Husbandry, Anjora, Durg (CG) from 2021 to 2022. She has received Young Scientist Award - 2019 from Agricultural and Environmental Technology Development Society (AETDS), U.S. Nagar, Uttarakhand during December 2019. She has published three research papers in national and international journals along with that more than 30 extension literature including popular articles, training mannuals, practical mannuals, book chapters, booklets, pamphlets, folders etc.

Practical Aspects in Veterinary Extension and Animal Husbandry

Ruchi Singh

Hari R.

Rashmi Vishwakarma

Manju Sahu

NIPA® GENX ELECTRONIC RESOURCES & SOLUTIONS P. LTD.

New Delhi-110 034

NIPA® GENX ELECTRONIC
RESOURCES & SOLUTIONS P. LTD.

101,103, Vikas Surya Plaza, CU Block
L.S.C.Market, Pitam Pura, New Delhi-110 034
Ph : +91 11 27341616, 27341717, 27341718
E-mail:newindiapublishingagency@gmail.com
www: www.nipabooks.com

For customer assistance, please contact
Phone: + 91-11-27 34 17 17 Fax: + 91-11- 27 34 16 16
E-Mail: feedbacks@nipabooks.com

ISBN: 978-93-91383-35-0

Composed and Designed by NIPA®.

Preface

As Veterinary Council of India (VCI) has revised the whole curricula of Bachelor of Veterinary Science and Animal Husbandry programme, there is requirement of students practical manual of Veterinary & Animal Husbandry Extension Education. In new pattern veterinary extension classifies in two parts, one for fundamental aspects of extension teaching (Paper-I, Unit-I) while another second part contain economics and entrepreneurship of livestock industry (Paper-II, Unit-II). An attempts has been made to give detailed information in systematic way like in the form of photographs, charts with supporting original field photographs to support the write up. For intricate analysis of the subject, in between experiment, a few exercise are given for practice of students which will help them in field exercise and their viva voce examination.

During compilation of this manual we have consulted various papers, test books, references book and internet sites from which so much guidance got it. So we are very thankful to all the esteemed scientists and authors whose book, bulletins, articles and sites we have consulted in the preparation of this book.

We also want to express my gratitude to my publishers who have made every effort to present the book in time.

Any suggestions for further improvement in the manual, from the academic fraternity and the students are most welcome. They would be taken note of and incorporated in next edition.

Authors

Contents

1

Collection and Analysis of Data

The word *data* means facts or information, specifically collected by the researcher through observation or measurement from which meaningful conclusions are drawn. Data may be of qualitative or quantitative types:

Qualitative **data** are descriptive/qualitative in nature and can be statistically analyzed only after processing and after having them classified into some appropriate categories.

Quantitative **data** are expressed in the form of numerals and are amenable to statistical analysis readily.

Primary **data** are those which are collected afresh and for the first time, specifically for the designated study.

Secondary **data,** on the other hand, are those which have already been collected and compiled by someone else.

There are many ways or tools for data collection. Some of them are as follows:

1. Interview schedule
2. Mailed questionnaire
3. Interview
4. Observation
5. Documentary sources

1. Interview schedule

The schedule is the form containing some questions or blank tables which are to be filled by the researchers after getting information from the respondents in face to face situation. This can also be done through telephonic conversations, video camera, tape recorder etc.

Advantages

1. This method is very useful in extensive enquiry and provide reliable results
2. It helps in getting first hand information
3. Retaining sequence of questioning
4. Personal contact is there, thus can clear any doubt at the spot.
5. Possible to study past phenomena

Limitations

1. The validity of data collected is always doubtful because of large number of sources of bias.
2. It is difficult task to a person agreeable for interview
3. For conducting an interview require a specialized knowledge of humane psychology and behavior.
4. It is more expensive to cover a wide area.

Difference between Interview Method and Questionnaire Method

Interview Method	Questionnaire Method
1. Researcher comes in direct contact with the respondent.	1. Direct contact with the respondent is not possible.
2. Data are collected directly in a face-to-face situation.	2. Data are collected indirectly through communication.
3. Questions are usually short.	3. Questions are rather lengthy to get detail information.
4. Data collected are more reliable.	4. Reliability of the data is somewhat doubtful.
5. A limited area can be covered.	5. A wide area can be covered.
6. Data can be collected from uneducated people by clarifying the meaning of questions.	6. Neither possible to clarify the questions, nor possible to get information from illiterate people.
7. A schedule is researcher-oriented.	7. A questionnaire is respondent-oriented.

2. Mailed questionnaire

In this method a questionnaire similar to the interview schedule is drafted. This questionnaire is then sent by mail to the respondents. They fill up the questionnaire and return it to the investigator.

Advantages

1. It is economical less expensive, reply can received in shorter time

2. It collected information from widely scattered area by literate people.

3. It can collect repetitive information at regular interval

Limitations

1. It cannot be applied for uneducated people

2. Some time respondents not send back the filled questionnaires

3. Lack of personal contact and information may not be reliable

3. Observation

Observation is probably the oldest method used by man in scientific investigation. There are three different types of observation. They are as follows.

1. Structured and Unstructured Observation: When observation is done on the basis of prefixed set of agenda and procedures it is called structured observation. When it is done on the basis of some ideas in mind about what, whom, how, where, and when to observe it is called unstructured observation.
2. Participant and Non-participant Observation: When the observer actively participates in the activity being observed it is called participant observation. But if he observes without an active participation in the activity being observed it is called non-participant observation.
3. Controlled and Non-Controlled Observation: When the observer has complete control on the subject being observed it is called controlled observation. Whereas, if he has little or no control on the subject being observed it is known as non-controlled observation.

4. Rating schedule

This type of schedule is used for sociological and psychological research. This is referred where attitude or opinion is to be measured. Different ranks or scale are constructed for this purpose. Ex: What is your opinion about vaccination in cattle?

i) Highly effective ii) Effective

iii) Not much effective iv) Not at all effective

5. Document schedule

This schedule is used for recording the data from already written documents like books, journal, office records, annual records, autobiography etc.

Social Survey

Broadly speaking there are two approaches for finding a solution to a given problem. They are Experimental Approach and Survey Approach. *Survey* is the systematic and comprehensive study of a set of people with a view to analyze a social problem and to recommend solution for that.

Social survey/survey research studies large and small *population/universe* by selecting and studying *sample* chosen from the *population/universe* to discover the relative incidence, distribution, and interrelations of *sociological* and *psychological variables*.

A social survey is a process by which quantitative and qualitative facts are collected about the social aspect of a community's composition and activities. Many research problems require the systemic collection of data from population or sample of population through the use of personal interview, questionnaire, observation, participatory interaction etc.

Type/ kinds of social survey

According to their subject matter, techniques of data collection, regularity etc. survey are classified in to four different types. They are as follows.

1. General and specific survey
2. Regular and ad-hoc survey
3. Preliminary and final survey
4. Census and sample survey

1. General or specific survey

When a survey is conducted for collecting general information about any population, institution or phenomena without any particular object or hypothesis is known as general survey. Ex. Census of livestock after every tenth year

Specific survey is conducted for specific problem or for testing the validity of some theory or hypothesis. Ex. Animal health services in rural area, Animal disease pattern in urban area.

2. Regular or ad-hoc survey

Some survey is regular in nature and must be repeated after regular interval. Such survey is undertaken where continuous data are required to study the trend or effect of time upon the phenomena under study. Ex. Family budget, rural credit survey of RBI

3. Preliminary or final survey

A preliminary survey generally known as 'pilot study' and it is the runner of the final survey. The purpose of this survey is to get the first hand knowledge of the universe to be surveyed. The final survey is made after the pilot survey.

4. Census and sample survey

In the census survey every single unit in the universe is to be contacted and information collected from him. In case of sample survey only a small part of it is taken as representative of the whole data. Ex. Census survey- Livestock census of the India

Sample survey - selection of few animals to know the breed characteristics

Utility of social survey in extension educational studies

- Social survey supply the information on any problem
- Survey is useful for testing the validity of many theories
- It explains the different causes behind the social problems
- It permits the researchers to come in direct contact with the people to whom he wants to study
- Survey method provides maximum reliable data of field condition from large number of respondents

Limitations of social survey

- Survey method is expensive, prolonged and time consuming
- The reliability and validity of the data depends upon the honest efforts done by the researchers
- Lack of in depth study

Exercise

Q.1 Conduct a social survey in your nearest village and collects information about cattle farming management practices

Q.2 Prepare an interview schedule in brief about adoption level of poultry farming practice?

2

Organizing Demonstration for Farmers

Demonstrations

Demonstration means showing by doing. The basic principle of Demonstration is learning by seeing and doing. The concept of demonstration was given by Dr. Seeman A. Knapp. Farmers like to see how a new idea works, both purposes can be achieved by means of a farm demonstration. A good, practical demonstration is an invaluable method in extension work. The demonstration is a particularly powerful method to use with farmers who do not read easily. There are two principal types of demonstration used by extension agents - method demonstration and result demonstration.

Method demonstration

- Method demonstrations basically show farmers how to do something. In the method demonstration, the farmer is shown step by step how. The agent will probably be dealing with farmers who have already accepted the particular practice being demonstrated, but who now want to know how to do it themselves.
- The main advantage of the method demonstration is that the extension agent can explain simple farming skills to a large number of people, thus increasing the impact of his extension work and the main limitation of a method demonstration is that, if there are too many farmers present, only a few get a chance to see, hear and do.

Result demonstration

- A result demonstration is an ideal way to present to farmers a comparison between traditional and new practices under local conditions. Comparison is the important element in a result demonstration: comparison between compost and no compost, between poor seed and selected seed, or between use of fertilizer and no fertilizer. "Seeing is believing" is an age-old expression, but one appropriate to a result demonstration.

Basic principles for demonstrations

- *Participation*
- *Simplicity*
- *Learning*
- *Preparation*
- During the demonstration, therefore, the agent should:
- ***Welcome*** the participants.
- ***Explain*** the purpose of the demonstration, what it is hoped to achieve and what the various stages are that will be followed.
- ***Conduct*** the demonstration in person or be ready to help the demonstrator farmer. Proceed at a pace the farmers can follow, and be prepared to explain again or answer questions from participants. Emphasize key points and explain the practice step by step in simple words.
- ***Summarize*** the main issues or points which have arisen, encourage questions from the farmers and make sure that the participants have had every opportunity to try out or examine the practice being demonstrated.
- ***Conclude*** the demonstration with a vote of thanks to all concerned, and with a few comments about any follow-up activities planned.

Follow-up

- This follow-up will be useful for the agent as well. Demonstrations can often result in good contacts with local farmers, and the agent may be able to enlist their support for future activities. The agent should, therefore, write a report and prepare a record of the demonstration.

3

Identification of Key Communicators by Socio-Metric Method

Identification of key communicators

For effective introduction of innovations and transfer of technology among farmers, effective communication is the prime need. An extension worker passes his information more effectively if he communicates with farmers/livestock owners through local leaders and key communicators.

Leader: Is a person who effectively influences a group to cooperate in setting and achieving the goal.

Leadership: Leadership is a process by which an individual influence, guide and direct the thought, feelings and impressions in desired way.

Key communicators: Key communicator is a person who has maximum information about his society and vicinity area on different aspects.

Need of local leader for extension work

The use of local leader is one of the unique differences between formal education and extension approach. Extension service development and expansion depends directly upon the degree of involvement of local leaders. The main purpose of identifying, development and utilization of rural leadership is to make available large number of teachers to teach farming community. It is impossible for any country to provide enough veterinarians, extension workers to carry information to each and every farmer at his doorstep. A local leader who has acquired the knowledge of improved practice extends the same to neighbour, friend and relatives. In any society and in every group in a community there are few individual who can influence other in the group and make decisions on behalf of other. They are the local leader. Most of the time the veterinarian is an outsider to the villagers. The people and their socio-culture pattern prevalent in that area may be new to him. Hence the local leader forms the vital link between the veterinarian and the livestock farmers. Hence, it is essential to identify and develop leadership that will facilitate and enhance effective working relationship with rural people.

Characteristics of Key Communicators

Key communicators' posses certain characteristics to a greater degree that set them apart from other farmers. Some of the important traits are.

- Popularity: They rank high in popularity status.
- Opinion leadership: Capable of influencing the decision and action of others.
- Progressivism: Highly receptive to modern values and practices.
- Scienticism: Do not give much importance to fate and luck.
- Venturesome: Not afraid of taking risk.
- Cosmopoliteness: Inclined to contact people outside his community.

Methods of Identification Key Communicators

Key communicators in a social system can be identified in a number of ways. Three methods are in common use.

- Socio-metric Method: In this method members of a social system are asked to name the person to whom they go for advice and information on a particular topic.
- Information Ratings: In this method some members of a social system are purposively or randomly selected and are asked to designate persons who are sought for advice and information by the fellow villagers.
- Self-designating Method: In this method each selected person is asked a series of questions designated to determine the degree to which he perceives himself to be a key communicator. Volunteers may be identified through this method.

Sociometry

Sociometry is a broad term indicating a number of methods of gathering and analyzing data on the choice, communication and interaction patterns of individuals in groups. Sociometry is the study and measurement of social choice. It has also been called a means of studying the attractions and repulsions of members of groups. There are three methods of Sociometric Analysis that are used for analysis of data collected through sociometric methods.

- Sociometric Matrices: A matrix is an array of numbers or symbols in rectangular form. Sociometric matrices are matrices of numbers expressing all the choices of members of the group studied. This is a convenient method of tabulation of sociometric data.

- Socio-grams: Socio-grams are diagrammatic representation of the internal structure of choices made by the members of a group.
- Sociometric Indices: Which are single numbers derived from sociometric data, which indicate the characteristics of individuals in the group. Groups in which members are known to each other should be selected for sociometric analysis.

Sociometric Matrices

In sociometry we are concerned with square, or n x n matrices, n being equal to the number of persons in a group. Rows of the matrix are labeled i; columns are labeled j. i and j can stand for any number and any person in the group. If we write a_{ij}, this means the entry in the ith row and jth column of the matrix, or more simply, any entry in the matrix.

Socio-gram

All the choices made by the group members can be depicted through socio-grams. From the data in Table, a socio-gram may be drawn. Here, a simple or one-way choice is represented by one-arrowed line like !, the mutual or two-way choice is represented by two-arrowed line like !. In case of no choice, no line exists. In preparing the socio-gram, the individual who has got maximum choice is put at the centre, followed gradually by others who have received lesser number of choices towards the periphery. To get a good socio-gram one may have to try out a number of diagrams.

An analysis of the sociometric data presented in the Table reveals the following information.

- B has received maximum number of choices in the group and is known as a star.
- BD and BH have received two-way or mutual choices.
- I, J and K received mutual choices, and form a tightly held sub-group which exclude other members of the group. This is a clique. Clique is defined as three or more individuals who mutually choose each other.
- CF form a mutual pair.
- AE, AB, HE and DH represent one-way choice.
- A received no choice, though he has given choice to others. Such individual is called rejectee.
- G has neither received nor made any choice. Such person is known as isolate.

These information may be depicted through socio-gram in the form of arrowed lines. So, from social action point of view, the socio-gram reveals that B is the most important person in the group or key communicator who must be contacted by an extension agent.

Socio-grams tell the investigator only which persons are chosen or rejected for a particular purpose, but do not provide any reason for their acceptance or rejection. For a deeper understanding of the sociometric choices it is necessary to compute some indices.

Sociometric Indices

In sociometry a large number of indices are possible. A simple but useful index is one which tells us about the choice status of an individual in the group. This is obtained by the equation

$$CS = \frac{\Sigma C}{n-1}$$

Where,

CS = Choice status of the person

ΣC = Sum of choices a person receives

n = Number of persons in the group

For example, choice status of B and C as per the Table

$$B = \frac{4}{11-1} = 0.40 \text{ or } 40 \text{ per cent}$$

$$C = \frac{1}{11-1} = 0.10 \text{ or } 10 \text{ per cent}$$

The value of choice status is the direct index of an individual's popularity in the group. This is also known as Sociometric Status Index. A measure of group cohesiveness may be obtained by the formula

$$CO = \frac{\Sigma(i \leftrightarrow j)}{\frac{n\,(n\text{-}1)}{2}}$$

$$CO = \frac{3}{\frac{3(3-1)}{2}} = 1.00 \text{ or } 100 \text{ per cent}$$

$$\frac{6}{11-1}$$

Where,

CO = Group cohesiveness

" (i ↔ j) = Sum of mutual choices or mutual pairs

n = Number of persons in the group

From the Table it may be found that there are six mutual pairs such as BH, BD, IJ, JK, KI and CF. Group cohesiveness of this group will be

$$CO = \frac{6}{\frac{11(11-1)}{2}} = 0.11 \text{ or } 11 \text{ per cent}$$

However, group cohesiveness of the clique in the given example represented by I, J and K will be

$$CO = \frac{3}{\frac{3(3-1)}{2}} = 1.00 \text{ or } 100 \text{ per cent}$$

It implies that the members who form clique are completely cohesive and may be treated as a singular body for social action.

Two more indices may be computed from the data in Table.

Social Compatibility Index is determined by the number of mutual choices (pairs) divided by one less than the group size. In the given example, the number of mutual choices is 6 and group size is 11.

$$\text{Social compatibility index of the group} = \frac{6}{11-1} = 0.60 \text{ or } 60 \text{ per cent}$$

Emotional Expansiveness is determined by the amount of utilization of available choices, expressed in percentage. From the Table it is seen that the sum total of choices made was (0 + 4 + 1 + 1 + 2 + 1 + 0 + 2 + 2 + 2 + 2) = 17 and the number of choices available are 22 (2 choices each for 11 members).

So, emotional expansiveness of the group = 17 / 22 x 100 = 77 per cent

Table: Sociometric matrix of an 11 member group with two choices (11x11 matrix)

								Chosen (j)		
A	**B**	**C**	**D**	**E**	**F**	**G**	**H**	**I**	**J**	**K**
	1	0	0	1	0	0	0	0	0	0
0		0	1	0	0	0	1	0	0	0
0	0		0	0	1	0	0	0	0	0
0	1	0		0	0	0	1	0	0	0
0	1	0	0		0	0	0	0	0	0
0	0	1	0	0		0	0	0	0	0
0	0	0	0	0	0		0	0	0	0
0	1	0	0	1	0	0		0	0	0
0	0	0	0	0	0	0	0		1	1
0	0	0	0	0	0	0	0	1		1
0	0	0	0	0	0	0	0	1	1	
Sum 0	4	1	1	2	1	0	2	2	2	2

Key communicator in a group may be identified by some another method such as

1. **Election:** In this method the group members will elect the leader. In the process of identification and right selection, the extension agent can help the people by explaining what sort of person is required to lead the group.
2. **Discussion method:** Through observation and discussion, the person with sound knowledge and ability is soon and easily recognized as leader.
3. **The workshop method:** Through this method, where large group breaks up into smaller groups and the responsibility of the programme and decision-making rest upon the smaller unit, leadership emerges in each group. The extension worker in the workshop has the position of consultant, observer, discussion group leader etc.
4. **Group observer method:** The extension worker should observe a group in action, which will enable him spot a potential leader. The group should not be aware of this.
5. **Key informant technique:** The veterinarian during his village visits can meet the key informants in a community and ask them to indicate the opinion of leader in their village.

Operating through Key Communicators/Volunteers in Society

Following are the means and ways of operating through key communicators and volunteers in society.

- The identified key communicators and volunteers may be approached and convinced personally.
- A good rapport may be developed by giving assurance and confidence by informing the purpose and nature of the programme.
- The identified key communicator and volunteers may be trained in a particular aspect of the programme which requires specific knowledge and skills.
- Group meeting and discussion may be conducted to give due recognition to them. Such meetings also provide an opportunity to group members in finding out common problems and their solutions. This will lead to the development of skill and habit of talking, thinking, planning and working together towards a common goal

Exercise

1. Draw a socio-gram for an imaginary group with choices showing mutual pairs, clique, star, etc.

4

Audio-Visual Equipments

"Audio-Visual aids are those instructional devices that may be used by a communicator in order to facilitate better understanding on the parts of learner by involving their many senses, particularly those relating to seeing and hearing".

As a potential link between research institutions and livestock owners the extension agent must have good skills in effectively communicating with various stakeholders which include policy makers, researchers, input suppliers, market agents, credit institutions etc.

Level of Retention

A study conducted by Hass and Packer (1964) showed that learning takes place through the various senses as under:

Sight	-	87.00%
Hearing	-	7.00%
Smelling	-	3.50%
Touch	-	1.50%
Taste	-	1.00%

Selection of Audio-Visual aids

The A.V. aids may be used singly or in combination with other aids in social sciences. The extension specialist should be well aware about the A.V. aids depending upon some factors which are as follows:

- Nature of subject matter
- Objectives of teaching
- Size of audience
- Audience nature: education, interest, age, experience, language etc.
- Availability of material, instruments, electricity, funds etc.

- Experience and skill of extension worker in making and utilization of A.V. aids

Features of A.V. aids: The important features of A.V. aids are as follows

- Provide the real picture of the topic
- Be in a good condition
- Be ideal and appropriate to intelligence or experience of learner
- Large number of aids should not be used together
- Best single or in combination to be selected
- Trainer should be able to use properly
- It must be worthy to time, expense and efforts involved

Advantages of A.V. aids

For communicating an idea, experience or technology, extension worker use audio-visual aids because audio-visuals help to communicate the message effectively and efficiently. They provide the audience with a situation nearest to the reality and readily get the idea. Research showed that the use of visual aids help people to learn faster and better than by verbal method, alone.

- Capture audience attention and arouse their interest
- Highlight main points of the message clearly
- The possibility of misinterpreting the concept is reduced
- Message perceived with several senses are easily understood and retained better
- The process and concepts that are expressed in words alone can be explained
- Develop continuity of thoughts
- Speed up the process of learning and bring effectiveness
- Can adopt the speed of presentation of the reactions of the audience
- Save time of teacher and learner

Classification of Audio-Visual Aids

There are many ways to classify Audio-Visual Aids. However the following classification system seems to be quite useful and adequate.

a) According to Evolution:

   i) First generation media: Handmade charts, graphs, exhibits, model etc.

ii) Second generation media: Printed/Illustrated text, work books etc.

iii) Third generation media: Photographs, slides, filmstrips etc.

iv) Fourth generation media: Television, computers etc.

b) According to Senses involved

i) **Audio-Aids:** These are those Instructional Aids through which messages can only be heard. e.g. Radio, Tape-recorder.

ii) **Visual Aids:** These are those Instructional aids through which messages can only be seen. e.g. Posters, Models.

1. Projected Aids: e.g. Slide Projector, OHP, Opaque Projector.
2. Non-Projected Display Aids: e.g. Posters, Models, Pictures.

iii) **Audio-Visual Aids:** These are those Instructional Aids through which messages can only be heard and seen. e.g. Television, Computer etc.

c) According to Type of Use

i) **Display type:** These are those devices that are spread before the audience for viewing, who then get the message by looking at them. E.g. Posters, Diagrams.

ii) **Presentation type:** These are those devices that are projected before the audience for viewing but at the same time one explains or presents the message of visuals so that the audience gets a meaningful understanding of them. E.g. Filmstrips, Flashcards etc.

Classification of Audio-Visual Aids

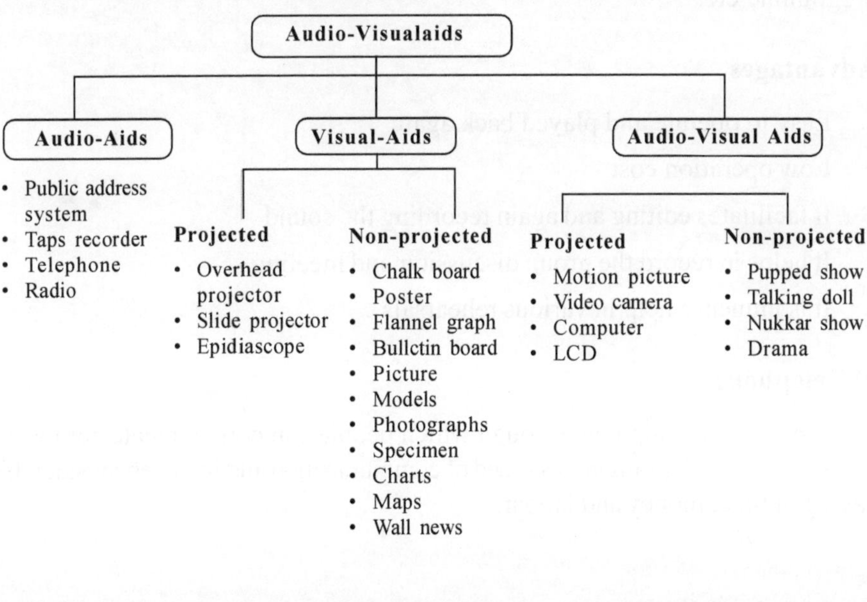

Audio Aids

a) Public address system (PAS)

It is a set of equipment to amplify the sound so that it is audible to a large audience over a distance. It is useful for extension programme involving a large number of people such as mass meeting, training programme, campaign, exhibition etc.

Component of public address system

- Microphone (mike)
- Amplifier and
- Loudspeaker

Resultant Impedance

When more than one Loudspeakers/Driver Units is connected in a combination to an amplifier, the combination has Resultant Impedance.

b) Tape recorder

It is equipment for recording sound on magnetic tape by electromagnetic process, which may be played back when needed. The tape may be of celluloid, plastic or high tensile polyester film. Tape has an ultra thin coating of iron oxide on one side. The tape is magnified as it passes through recording head. Tape recorder is suitable for use in meeting, training programme, campaign, recording radio programme etc.

Advantages

- Easy to operate and played back again
- Low operation cost
- It facilitates editing and again recording the sound
- It helps in record the group discussion and meeting.
- It is immense help in various rehearsals.

c) Telephone

It is a system of equipment through which people can communicate both ways to distant places. This improves speed of communication and involves considerable saving of time, money and labour.

d) Radio

Radio is one of the oldest and popular IT tools and provides extensive information to farmers. It is an electronic audio medium for broadcasting programmes for audience. This medium is cosmopolite in approach and is suitable for communication to millions of people widely dispersed and situated in remote areas. At present, the broadcasting network in India covers about 93% of the population, spread over 82 percent of geographical area.

Advantages

- Radio has the advantage of being able to bring the first hand experience of an authority on a subject within the reach on every radio listener.
- This medium commands a universal audience by geographic spread, income, education, age, and sex etc. and thus reaches an audience not often reached by other mass media.
- Education through radio is inexpensive compared to other methods.
- Radio is suitable for creating general awareness amongst the people, help change their attitude and reinforces learning.
- The medium is extremely convenient for communication at time of crisis and urgent situation.
- It reaches a large number of people at very low cost.
- The programme can be listening while audience engaged in other work.

Visual Aids: (Non-Projected)

1. Chalk board

The chalkboard popularly known as black board is most universally used teaching aid. It is board for writing with chalk. The chalk board is probably the simplest, cheapest, most convenient and widely used visual aid. For field use, inward folding wooden board or roll-up material can be used in lecture, training programme, group meeting etc.

2. Bulletin board

Bulletin board is a board for display of message which may be fixed by board-pin on the soft insulation board. The message on the bulletin board may be in the form of words, graph, charts, photographs, publication etc. It helps to draw attention to important announcements and high light current activities and achievements.

3. Picture and photograph

Picture is a representation made by drawing, painting or photograph, which gives accurate idea of an object. Picture may be black and white or in colour. They are used in various ways such as training programme, farm publication, campaign, exhibition slide etc.

4. Flannel graph, Flash card, Flip chart

Flannel graph, Flash card and Flip chart are visual aids in which the message are written or drawn on thick paper and presented step by step by the extension agent to the audience to synchronize with talk. This produces a dramatic effect on the audience.

5. Poster

Poster is visual aid and display in a public place for the purpose of creating awareness amongst the people. A poster is generally seen at a distance.

A poster should have the corresponding properties

- It must be able to attract the attention
- It must convey the message quickly
- It must lead to action

6. Diagram, Map, Chart and Graph

These are visual aids where information is summarized and presented in a more or less abstract form

- **Diagram** is line drawing of an object or an idea.
- **Map** is an informative diagram of an area
- **Chart** contains information in tabular form
- **Graph** is a diagrammatic representation of the relationship between variables

Diagram, Map, Chart and Graph are used in bulletin board, method demonstration, group meeting, training programme, farm publication, exhibition etc.

7. Specimen, model and diorama

- **Specimen** is a sample, which represents the whole.
- **Model** is a miniature replica of an object.
- **Diorama** is a scenic representation of the original, with specimen, model, and painting.

8. Translides

These are transparent big size photograph, which are display by providing light at the back. For this purpose, shallow wooden boxes are made with front side open and backside fixed on wall with hinge.

Visual Aids (Projected)

1. Slide

Slide is a mounted picture, which is projected by focusing light through it. Projection is made by slide projector on roll back screen or on white wall. Slide of 35 mm films mounted on cardboard or plastic frames are more common.

2. Filmstrip

It is a continuous strip of films consisting of number of individual frame or picture arranged in a sequence. Each strip may contain about 30 to 60 frame of photograph, diagrams, drawing or lettering. The entire length of strip has perforation on both sides, which facilitate forward and back ward movement of the pictures.

3. Opaque projector or epidiascope

Opaque projector is a large aperture projector and used to project opaque materials. It is also known as epidiascope. Picture, drawing, diagram directly from the book can be projected. This type of projector works on the principle of reflected projection.

4. Overhead projector (OHP)

In O.H.P. the picture is projected over the head of the speaker on the screen. Drawing, diagram, lettering etc. are made on transparent sheets and are put on the glass platform of the over head projector through which strong light is passed.

Audio-Visual Aids (Non-Projected)

1. Drama

Drama is a theatrical performance around a theme by some people who have rehearsed for it.

2. Puppet show

The doll is made to perform by control movement of the puppeteer from outside. Both the media require adequate preparation and rehearsing. Puppet may be different type glove or hand puppets, string puppets, rod puppets and shadow puppets.

3. Talking Doll

Talking doll is an innovation and may be used to create general awareness of a group of people about an extension programme. Its use is, however, restricted to the availability of an expert ventriloquist, who cannot project own voice, but is also able to manipulate the movement of the doll to synchronize with the voice.

Drama, puppet show and talking doll provide dramatic experience to the audience and may be used to communicate message on broad social themes pertaining to the rural life, rather than transfer of technology programmes.

Audio-Visual Aids (Projected)

1. Motion picture (Cinemas)

Motion picture is the projected image of positive print of a sound film taken by a movie camera, which produces synchronized movement of picture with sound. The film consist of series of still pictures, which when projected on a screen in rapid succession, produce the optical illusion of a continuous picture in which object appear to move. The films may be of 16 mm, 35 mm, and 70 mm width. The film with 16 mm width is generally used in extension work.

Video: It is an electronic audiovisual system for preparing videotapes of programmes and events, which could be projected through their receiving set with moving images and synchronized sound. This is useful in repeated presentation, but involves technical skill in production.

2. Computer multimedia

It brings together, text, graphics, animation, video still image, and audio and motion video. It is a strong teaching tool, uses all their sense and enables learner to hear and see.

3. Folk media

A communication system embedded in the culture which existed before the arrival of mass media, and still exists as a vital mode of communication in many parts of the world, present in community despite of certain degree of change. To a society, folk media are culturally more compatible.

Recent extension communication Methods

Satellite Communication

The first experiment with satellite television broadcasting was conducted in India in 1975-76 when the Satellite Instructional Television Experiment (SITE) was launched.

Internet

It is an international computer network connecting other networks and computers from Company, Universities etc. It enables the people to access vast global information resources. It can facilitate dialogue among communities, planners, development agencies, researchers and technical experts and encourage community participation in decision-making.

Multimedia

Multimedia describes the use of different media and technologies to present the information in variety of ways. It is a multifaceted instructional strategy that brings together text, graphics, animation, video, still images, audio and motion video. Computer multimedia is a strong teaching tool since it facilitates more complete use of learner senses in a learning situation. This technology can help extension workers and scientist to integrate modeling visualization and decision making process associated with various farming systems.

Video Conferencing

It is an audio plus visual conferencing for farmers located in distance villages through World Wide Web (WWW). Extension work can choose the programme as they wish during the entire period stipulated by them. This technology is very flexible and open to entire world.

Teleconferencing

It is the interaction between the individuals of groups through satellite television. It is an advance electronic aid by which we can exchange latest technologies available in different countries. It can be effectively carried out with the help of geocentric satellites send by different countries.

Compact Disc-Read Only Memory (CD-ROM)

The Compact Discs or Optical Discs are the alternative to the magnetic tapes. A CD-ROM can store large amount of information in compact and convenient form.

Expert System

This system provides ready access to information to extension personal and farmers. This new technologies provides advice and information immediately to user. This system gives an opportunity to see that how A.H. / agriculture experts are capable in solving day-to-day problems of the farmers.

Geographical Information System

The Geographical information System is a computer-based data bank for the information generated through remote sensing which is stored and preserved in the raw as well as processed form. It is a power full tool for data management and helps in natural resource management and sustainable animal husbandry and agricultural development.

5

Principle and Use of Projectors

Overhead Projector

Principles of Over Head Projector (OHP)

A projector, which projects the image over the head of an instructor on the screen, is called OHP. It worked on the principle of indirect projection. With the use of lens of short focal length and two mirrors the picture is reflected on the screen. The drawing, diagram, letter (may be in colour or in black and white) etc. are made on transparent sheet and are put on the glass platform of the OHP, through which strong light is passed. The rays of light are converged by a lens and reflected by a mirror held at an angle of 45°.

Over Head Projector

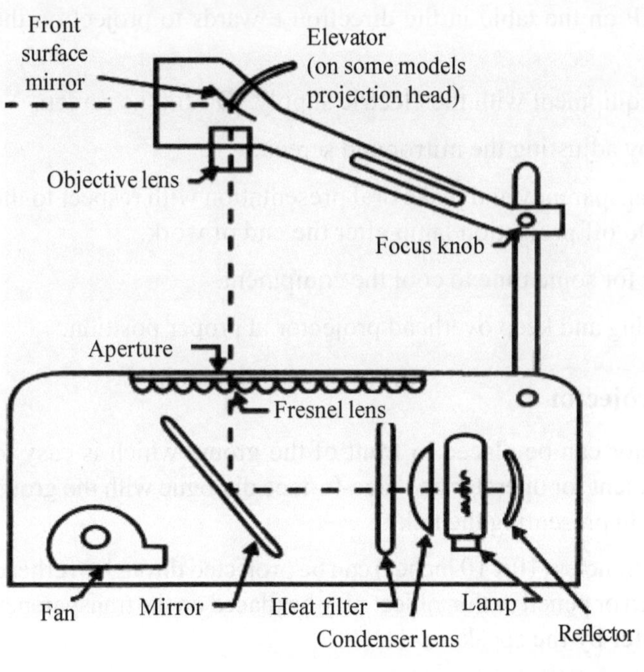

Functions of important parts of overhead projector

1. Lamp- A tungsten halogen lamp that is the source of light. (600 Watt; 240 V), it produces a light from its filament, which is arranged along the axis of projection.
2. Objective lens- It is fixed with lens holder
3. Heat filter- it absorbs the infrared rays from the lamp and prevent overheating.
4. Mirror- it is set at 45° angle to the axis of the preceding part, which reflects light into a vertical axis to the lens.
5. Focusing knob- it adjusts raise or lower the projection head to get clear image on the screen.
6. Glass stage-: The glass plate on which the OHP transparency is placed.
7. Control knob- it controls the supply of light.
8. Arm- it is horizontal to glass stage and hold objective lens.
9. Condenser Lens: It evenly distributes the glass stage placed above it and also converges the beams to the Projection Lens.

Handling of overhead projector

- Do keep the OHP on the table in the direction towards to project on the screen.
- Do connect the equipment with the electric supply. Do fix the screen.
- Do clear image by adjusting the mirror and screen.
- Do project the transparency and make oral presentation with respect to the written matter. Do off projection lamp after the end of work.
- Do allow the fan for some time to cool the equipment.
- Do remove the plug and keep overhead projector at proper position.

Use of overhead projector

1. Overhead projector can be placed in front of the group, which is easy to handle the equipment for operator and face-to-face dialogue with the group and it saves time in presenting the talk
2. Large size transparencies (10 x 10 inches) can be projected through overhead projector and a pen or pencil or thin object may be placed on the transparency and used as pointer by the speaker.

3. It can project various kinds of teaching aids viz. charts, graphs, drawings, diagrams, maps and worksheets which are prepared in transparent materials like sheets of plastic or cellophane paper to write or draw sketches on them a special type of ceramic pencil or crayon (marker) is used for this purpose e.g. Master Vu-graph OHP.
4. It is used in training programs, group meetings, seminar, symposium and workshop etc.

Slide Projector

Principle of slide projector

Slide projector is based on the principle of direct projection. In slide projector when light falls on a transparent object, it passes through the object. If the light is made to pass through a convex lens and allowed to fall on a screen at a convenient distance, an inverted image of the object will appear on the screen. If the object is initially kept inverted before the source of light the image will be straight and comprehensible.

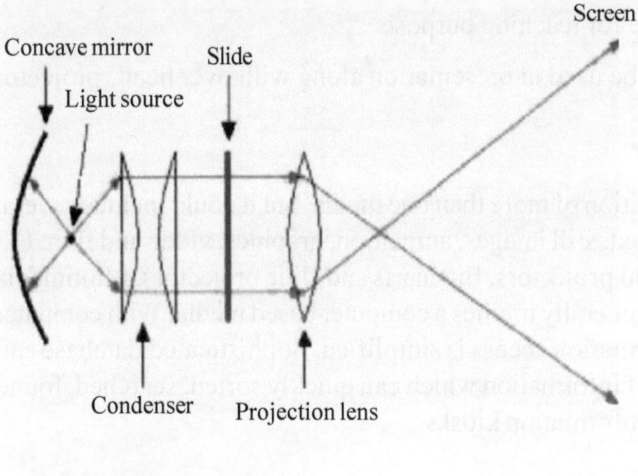

Parts of Slide Projector

A. Optical Parts

1. Projection Lamp: To reflect the light towards the condenser.
2. Reflecting Concave Mirror: To project light evenly over the object to be projected.
3. Condenser: To condense the reflecting light.
4. Projection Lens Barrel: For projecting the image on the screen.

B. Mechanical Parts

1. Cooling Fan: Keep the Projection Lamp House cool by blowing air.
2. Tilt Screw: To adjust the projector at the desired level.
3. Framer: For adjusting the film on the frame.
4. Lock Pin: To bring the vertical frame to a horizontal position and vice-versa.
5. Film-strip carrier: To carry the film strip
6. Slide Carrier: To carry the slides
7. Slide Carrier Lock
8. 3- Position Switch: Controls the cooling fan and Projection Lamp.

Use of slide projector

1. For slide projector, required slides (2" x 2") can be made easily, quickly and practically no cost by using local material
2. Slide projector can be used in seminars, workshops, conferences or educational institute for teaching purpose.
3. Slide projector can be used in presentation along with over head projector

Multimedia Projector

Multimedia is a combination of more than one media, but it could include several forms of media-audio, text, still images, animation, graphics, video and film. Ex: Combination of overhead projectors, flipcharts and slide projectors. Multimedia is more current context generally implies a computer based media. With computer based multimedia, information access is simplified. Sophisticated database can organize vast amounts of information which can quickly sorted, searched, found and cross indexed. Ex: information kiosks

Advantages

1. It enhances the effect of text presentations and improves the quality of presentation and retains the attention of audience.
2. It is good for use on computers.
3. It can be used for educational as well as entertainment purpose.
4. Multimedia presentations can be modified very easily.
5. It is quick and easier to operate for the instructor.

C. Digital Video/ Still Camera

"Photography is the art, science, and practice of creating pictures by recording radiation on a radiation-sensitive medium, such as a photographic film, or electronic image sensors"

Principle of working Digital Video or Still Camera

Photography uses foremost radiation in the UV, visible and near-IR spectrum. For common purposes the term light is used instead of radiation. Light reflected or emitted from objects form a real image on a light sensitive area (film or plate) or a FPA pixel array sensor by means of a pin hole or lens in a camera during a timed exposure. The result on film or plate is a latent image, which is developed into a visual image (negative or diapositive). An image on a paper base is known as a print.

Still photography

Refers to the art of producing still images. This is done with the help of simple or digital camera.

"A digital camera (or digicam) is a camera that takes video or still photographs, or both, digitally by recording images via an electronic image sensor."

Uses

1. Photography is used by extension workers for demonstrations, preserve and record memories of important events, to capture special moments, to tell stories, to send messages.
2. Convenience of sending images by email, placing them on the World Wide Web, or displaying them in digital picture frames.
3. Photography has many uses for business, science, manufacturing (Photolithography), art, and recreational purposes.

Exercise

Q.1 Draw a labeled diagram of Over Head Projector.

Q.2 Draw a labeled diagram of slide projector.

Q.3 Write down the definition, use and principle of Slide Projector.

Q.4 What is multimedia projector? Write down its importance.

6

Preparation of Radio Script

Radio script should be prepared in such a way that listener should feel that somebody is talking with him in a friendly manner and with informal style. For this purpose:

1. Collect the material from your experience.
2. Keep the purpose of the script and audience in mind.
3. Decide the method of presentation of information.
4. Considering the time available for the talk, the script should be prepared.
5. Generally we talk two words per seconds and 8 to 10 lines are required per minute having 5-6 words per sentences.
6. Time for talk is always limited hence select one idea at a time never include maximum technical information in the script.
7. Arrange the information in the sequences.
8. Include supporting and illustrated facts.
9. See that audience can understand your talk, for that use short an simple sentence, familiar words and personal words like I we, You.
10. Never use statistical table in a dialogue.
11. Repeat where ever necessary to emphasis the important points. At the end summaries the main point.

Exercise

Q.1 Prepare one script for radio talk based on animal husbandry.

6

Preparation of Radio Script

Radio script should be prepared in such a way that listener should feel that somebody is talking with him in a friendly manner and with informal style. For this purpose:

1. Collect the material from your experience.
2. Keep the purpose of the script and audience in mind.
3. Decide the method of presentation of information.
4. Considering the time available for the talk the script should be prepared.
5. Generally one talk two words per seconds and 8 to 10 lines are required per minute having 15-20 words per sentences.
6. Time for talk is always limited hence select one idea at a time never include too much technical information in the script.
7. Arrange the information in the sequences.
8. Include supporting and illustrated facts.
9. See that audience can understand your talk for that use short and simple sentence, familiar words and personal words like I, we, you.
10. Never use statistic (data) in the dialogue.
11. Repeat whenever necessary to emphasis the important points. At the end summaries the main point.

Exercise

Q. 1. Prepare the script of radio talk based on your background.

7

Preparation of Television Script

TV Talk

The talk delivered through TV i.e. through an electronic audio-visual medium which provides pictures with synchronized sound. The medium is cosmopolite in nature and can be used to develop instant mass awareness.

Important points while writing a programme for broadcasting

- Writing should be catchy, readable, conversational sound, understood and absorbed by the audience.
- Writing should be in simple, known language avoiding too much technicalities
- Interest of the listener should be sustained continuously
- Application of figures should be done judiciously
- Preparation of outline and arrangement in reasonable sequence
- Rehearsing the radio talk before deliberation, make sure that content and treatment are adequate to convey the message
- Farmers do value to variety, novelty and emotional touch and pitch in your voice.

1. Importance of television

- Most powerful media of mass communication because of audio and visual aids.
- Cover more audience
- Education with entertainment
- Audio as well as visual

2. Krishi darshan programme telecast from Mumbai(1967)

3. Present T. V. programme in India

- DD-KISHAN special channel for agriculture

- GRAM-JAGAT
- KRUSHI DARSHAN
- ANNADATA
- KHETINI VAAT

Doordarshan was started in April 1,1976

First T.V. station was established at Delhi (1965).

Steps for preparing script for T.V. programme

1. Selection of subject matter.
2. Select an Appropriate topic from selected subject.
3. Determine main points of selected topic.
4. Get overall picture of programme in mind.
5. Divide into important steps and arrange in logical order.
6. Consult resource person for advise.
7. Selection of format or method of presentation.
8. Determine the participants.
9. List out all the visual, equipment and material to be used.
10. Make an outline of programme.
11. Correct out line as per suggestion of programme producer.
12. Prepare audio to each segment according to time segment
13. Rehearse programme and add or subtract materials to fit the script into the desired time.
14. Decide time segment according to its important in programme.
15. Decide background music or Falk dance for programme.

8

Preparation and Use of Poster and Chart

Principle of construction of poster making

A poster is to be bold in design, simple to understand and attractive in colour. Poster is displayed in a public place with the purpose of creating awareness amongst the people. A poster is generally seen from a distance and the person glancing at to get first idea about it. Construction of poster making should be based on following components.

1. Pictures
2. Words
3. Space
4. Colors
5. Layout

a) Picture or illustration

1. Picture should be drawn in such a way that produce message clearly.
2. Avoid unnecessary details so that viewer's attention will not be diverted.
3. While preparing illustrations, experiences of people should be kept in mind as well as used objects must be familiar to them.

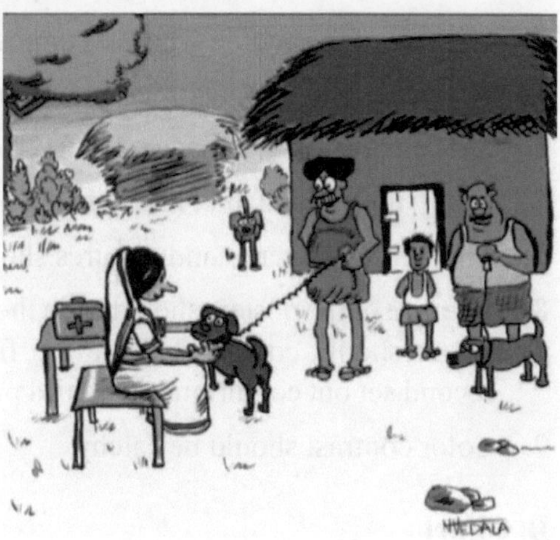

b) Caption in words Vaccinate your animals first

1. Five words caption is the best.
2. Caption should be written horizontally which helps in easy reading

c) Colour

1. Use bright and attractive colors.
2. Do not use more than three colors to avoid confusion of readers.

d) Space

1. Poster should not be loaded with pictures and words.
2. Adequate space should be provided to make clarity.

e) Layout

It should be well balanced so that viewer's eyes can run smoothly and quickly through caption and illustration.

Following points are to be kept in mind in preparation of Posters

It must always be a part of a campaign or a teaching programme and should be followed with other devices such as meeting, demonstrations etc.

1. A good poster arouses or urges people to immediate action and is highly suggestive.
2. It carries one idea at a time for a special job.
3. It is meant for people who are supposed to do the job.
4. It should be attractive, brief and clear. (ABC of Poster making)
5. It tells the story at a glance, letters should be bold.
6. Easily understandable, readable from a distance of about 15-20 meters.
7. The written material and pictures should be balanced.
8. The size of the posters should be in the ratio of 2:3, preferably 20"x30". The poster should contain 3 parts- the first part announces the purpose, the second set out conditions, and third part recommend action.
9. Color contrast should be catchy.

B. Chart

A chart is a visual symbol summarizing or comparing or contrasting or performing other helpful services in explaining subject matter. A chart contains series of ideas. While a poster is generally used in the awareness stage, a chart is used in the later stages especially in the testing stage either alone or in combination with the other aids.

Types of chart

Flip chart: Flip chart carries a series of ideas arranged sequentially. Individually charts tagged or bound to some support. During teaching these flips are turned one by one in a sequence.

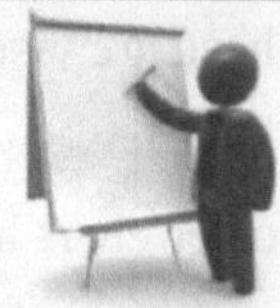

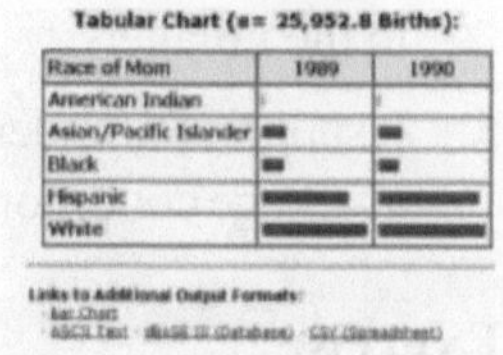

Tabular chart: Anything that is recorded or presented in a tabular form is a tabular chart.

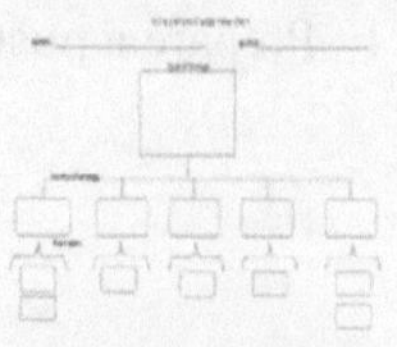

Flow chart: These are made by lines, arrows, rectangles etc. They show the structure of an organization, institution, association etc. It can also be used to show the story of a product as to how it has been obtained through a series of processes.

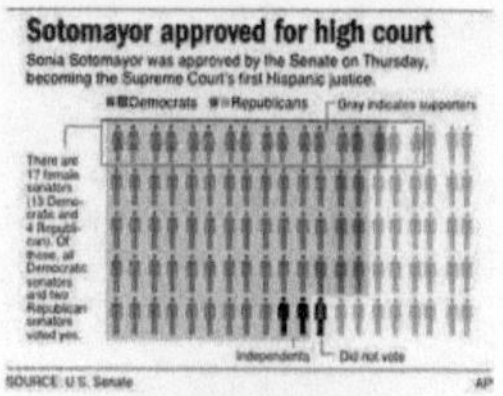

Pictorial chart: A chart may contain pictures suitably coloured & written matter. It may also contain a graph or may be a combination of pictures and graphs.

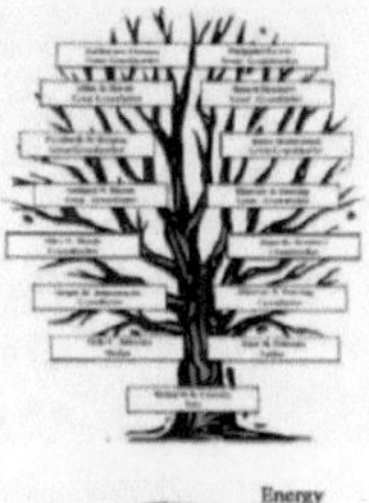

Tree chart: These are used to show development or growth of things. In this the origin is a single line. The various developments are shown as branches.

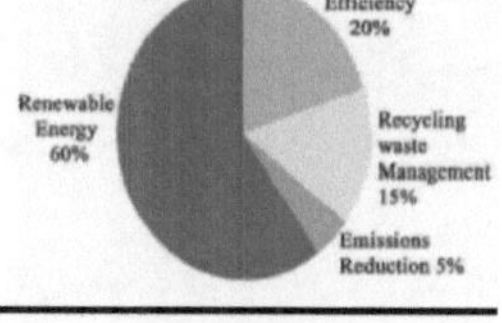

Pie chart/graph: These are in the shape of circles and used to show how several parts make up the whole. Each section should have its own colour and the size based on the section proportion.

Pull chart: The content of the chart is put fully in suspense by placing another sheet of paper of the same size with the help of two paper clips.

Strip roll up chart: In this type of chart, the points are recorded on series of strips, rolled up in sequences and displayed in order on a big size of paper. This type of chart leads to dramatic effect. It helps the trainer to develop the lesson systematically.

Use of poster/chart

1. These are visual non-projected aid used for teaching purpose.
2. These have wide approach to educate livestock farmers.
3. Poster/chart helps the extension worker to get an idea to the audience.
4. Poster/chart has long durability of presentation, which serves as a reminder to the villagers.
5. It support for understanding of farmers during demonstrations and exhibitions at village condition.

Exercise

Q.1 Prepare a poster/chart based on animal husbandry.

9

Preparation and Use of Flash Card Flannel Graph and Flip Chart

Principle of construction of flash cards

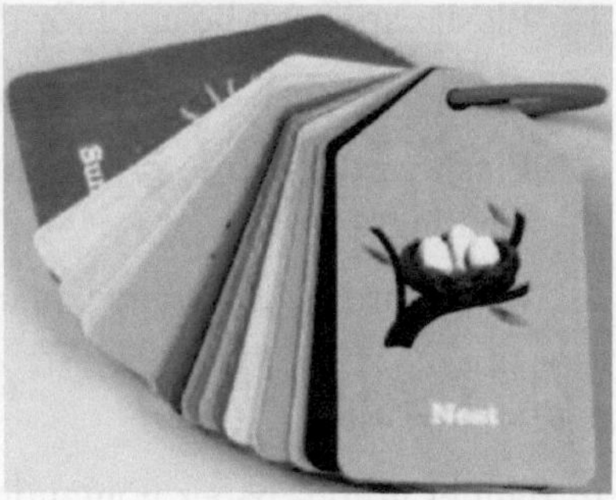

- Flash cards are non-projected visual aid in which series of illustrated cards are flashed as presented in a proper sequence to explain complete story.
- The story must be familiar, with specific heading and suggestions at the last.
- Simple words and local expressions should be used in flash cards.
- Total number of flash cards must be 10 -12 which are easy to remember to farmers
- Card: Select white or light coloured thick paper.
- Flash card should be large enough for everyone to see at least 22 x 28 inches and simple line drawing or photographs or cartoons having plenty of colours.
- Content: Each set should have a title card. The story should be divided into a number of scenes, which are to be presented in number of individual cards. Each card must have message, presented in simple line drawing, photographs, cartoons, and cutouts with few words.
- Lettering: Have lettering large enough for the group to read. At least 1" high.
- Colours: Use dark colours. But not more than three colours.
- Words: Use minimum words, not more than 10 to 12 words per card.

Presentation

1. The speaker must familiar with the story for each card.
2. Arrange the card in their proper sequence.
3. As one card is finished, slip the front card to the back of the set.
4. After the story is completed, display the card on a bulletin board or pass them on to interested person, if needed.
5. Use this card along with other teaching aids.

Use of flash card

1. Flash cards can be used for the group not more than 30 people.
2. Flash cards can be adapted to local conditions.
3. Flash cards help to create interest among illiterate farmers during group meetings.
4. Flash cards can be made quickly because of inexpensive local materials.

Flannel Graph

In flannel graph, paper containing the message is prepared with sand paper backing and is placed one by one in a sequence along with talk, on a board cover with flannel or hand woven thick cloth (khaddar graph).

Flip Chart

Flips carry a series of ideas arranged sequentially. Individually charts are tagged or bound to some support. During teaching, these flips are turned one by one in a sequence.

Exercise

Q.1 Prepare flash cards which can communicate a message through a small story having concept of animal husbandry.

10

Preparation and Use of Farm Publications for Extension Work

A. Circular letter

- Circular letter is a quick and cheap method of communication.
- It is a letter reproduced and sent to many people by the extension worker, to publicize an extension activity (like meeting, exhibits etc.) or to give information on farm and home problems.
- Circular letter could be used as a mail before organizing any campaign or extension work.
- It is sent from extension wing weekly or fortnightly to maintain regular contact with the farmers depending upon the need of time and facilities available in the field.

B. Advisory letter

- Advisory letters are generally written to advice the farmers.
- Advisory letters contents advice in the form preliminary information like prevention and control of diseases by vaccination of animals.
- The same text of advisory letter can be sent to number of farmers.
- Advisory letters have an importance of time and season.

C. Leaflet

- It is a single sheet of paper used to present information on only one topic in a concise manner with simple language. e.g. package of practices for prevention and control of disease.
- It can be used mostly in urban areas.
- If leaflet contain illustrations which become easy to get an idea to illiterate farmers in rural area.

D. Folder

Folder is a single sheet of paper folded ones or twice when it is opened; the material presented is in sequence. In folder, there is no need to write the complete sentence as paragraph. Folder can be made attractive by different photographs or illustrations. It can be used for large number of farmers at the time of group meetings or exhibitions.

E. Bulletin

It is a printed farm publication in the form of bound booklet with a number of pages containing comprehensive message relating to essential topics. A small piece may be taken for some valuable bulletins and prepared as and when required.

F. Journal, Magazine

This periodical also indicates different achievements and activities of our society published by some organizations or institutes. It contains different types of information associated with various topics of interest not only for the villages but also for extension workers. This is normally given against prepayment of subscription to the members for a particular period and has a fixed periodicity of publication.

Exercise

Q.1 Write the names of any 5 journals based on animal husbandry.

11

Planning and Organizing an Awareness Campaign (Health and Production)

Awareness campaign should help educate your community on a specific subject by sharing basic information and providing examples. This will help community members have healthy conversations and increase awareness. This will begin the prevention process. Any awareness campaign should include following step;

1. Choose Your Topic Or Goals
2. Find Your Resources: Awareness campaigns take a lot of resources. You might have a set budget to implement your campaign. Money is not the only resource you will be using. Resources such as time, marketing and promotional material etc also needed for successful completion of campaign.
3. Segment Your Audience
4. Create a Schedule of Events, Programs, and Initiatives
5. Once you have your goals, know your resources and audience, you can plan the specific events of your awareness campaign. The type of events you put on should build from your goals, resources, and audiences to include various active and passive awareness campaigns.
6. A passive campaign method uses promotional materials or handouts to bring awareness and education on a specific topic.
7. An active campaign method may use educational sessions that present information directly to individuals and are designed to reach multiple groups.
8. Create Action Plans for the Campaign: The general idea of planning should answer the questions who, what, where, when, why and how.
9. Find Partners
10. Implement Action Plan
11. Evaluate The Campaign

12. Continue Ongoing Awareness: One of the best ways to carry-out your campaign during the year is to continue to host similar events or provide education to make awareness of the issue part of your community. Another option is to create new ways of engaging community members, keeping track of their information, and building a list of who might be willing to volunteer with future events.

12

Planning and Organization of Animal Health Camps

The following is the plan of action to hold Animal Health Camps

1. Attempt will be made to hold at Gram Panchayat level.
2. Before 2-3 days monadi of camps must be do.
3. The camp will be held for 1 day. It will start by 7 AM and close at 2 PM.
4. The venue should be selected so that it is in the central location to get cases from 3-4 villages in order to provide facilities of clinical examination, pathological tests, etc.
5. The venue should be centrally located and easily accessible to the general public.
6. Selection of venue should be done in consultation with the local members, MPCS and CDVO/SDVO.
7. The camp will provide health care services along with awareness and information at the doorsteps of the people for promoting preventive, curative veterinary services.
8. Special focus would be on reducing infertility problems in dairy cow and to induce heat through controlled breeding programme.
9. Approximately, 50 dairy animals will be treated for reproductive disorders and 50 animals will be treated for other ailments in the camp.

13

Exercise on Rapid Rural Appraisal (RRA) and Participatory Rural Appraisal (PRA) Technique

'Extension' acts as a potential link between 'research' and 'teaching' which also facilitates transfer of technology. In this context new concepts, like Rapid Rural Appraisal (RRA) and Participatory Rural Appraisal (PRA) are becoming more meaningful now-a-days.

Rapid Rural Appraisal (RRA)

i) RRA can be defined as a systematic but semi-structured study, carried out in the field by a multi-disciplinary team over a short period ranging from three days to three weeks, based on information collected in advance from published and/or unpublished sources, direct observations and interviews as to generate working hypotheses for subsequent action

ii) RRA study aims at generating information on rural life and conditions that is relevant, timely, accurate and usable in a cost-effective way. It is based on the principle of participation and offers a range of methods, both existing ones and adapted and new ones.

Participatory Rural Appraisal (PRA)

i) It comprises a set of techniques aimed at shared learning between local people and outsiders. PRA is learning through participation about livelihood system and interaction of various facts. It helps in joint evaluation of problems and opportunities.

ii) PRA is intended to enable people to conduct and share their own investigations and analysis.

iii) RRA and PRA are not clearly defined. They have evolved from, draw on, and resonate with several other approaches such as Farming Systems Research, Participatory Action Research and Agro-ecosystem Analysis.

There are different types of participatory methods and tools/techniques of data collection. They are as follows.

1. **Space-related PRA Methods**: These methods are useful for exploring the spatial dimension of people's realities. The focus is on how people perceive and relate to space rather than just to the physical aspects as they exist. They include various types of participatory mapping, e.g. social mapping, resource mapping, mobility mapping, transect mapping, census mapping, etc.
2. **Time-related PRA Methods**: These methods help in exploring the temporal dimensions of people's realities. They allow people to use their own concept of time while describing or explaining an incident, phenomenon, etc. They are time line, trend analysis, daily activity schedule, seasonal diagram, etc.
3. **PRA Relation Methods:** PRA uses similar guidelines and tools to RRA but focuses on the stimulation of participation by local people. Specific techniques are used to encourage greater involvement among people and to enable them to take the leading role in appraising conditions and identifying solutions. The role of the PRA team is to make itself unnecessary as quickly as possible. They include cause-effect diagram, Venn diagram/chapatti diagram, ranking methods (pair wise ranking, wealth ranking, matrix ranking), pie diagram, etc.

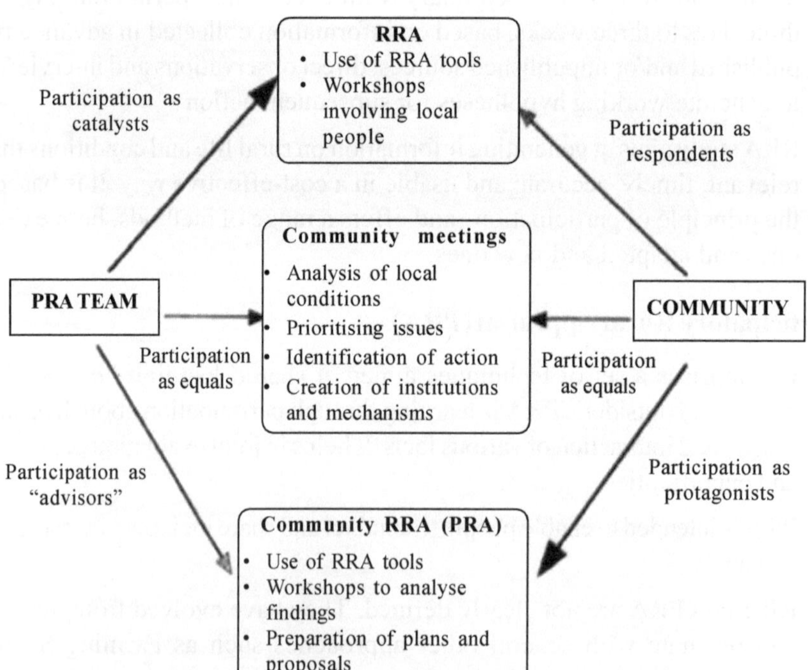

PRA Process

Other PRA methods that are not included in the above types are listing, semi-structured interview, topical interview, key informant interview, focus group interview, observation, etc.

Potential Differences between RRA and PRA

RRA	PRA
Responding to needs of development workers and agencies	Responding to needs of communities and target groups
More emphasis on efficient use of time & achievement of objectives	More emphasis on flexibility to adapt to time frame of community
Communication and learning tools used to help outsiders analyse conditions and understand local people	Communication and learning tools used to help local people analyse their own conditions and communicate with outsiders
Focus of RRA decided by outsiders	Focus of PRA decided by communities
End product mainly used by development agencies and outsiders	End product mainly used by community
Enables development agencies and institutions to be more "participatory"	Enables (empowers) communities to make demands on development agencies and institutions
Can be used purely for "research" purposes without necessarily linking to subsequent action or intervention	Closely linked to action or intervention and requiring immediate availability of support for decisions and conclusion s reached by communities as a result of the PRA

Strategy and methodology for working

i) The use of a variety of data collection methods means different kinds of information can be obtained. Validity or trustworthiness of the data is sought by intense and prolonged engagement with the local people, systematic cross checking of information (by use of multiple sources of information, use of varying techniques and alternative working hypothesis) and periodic meetings of the research group in which reality is viewed from varying angles or disciplines and alternative working hypothesis are developed, analyzed and compared and/or integrated.

ii) The professionals should facilitate investigation, analysis, presentation and learning by the local (rural or urban) people themselves. The researcher has to establishing good rapport with the local population and functions first and for all as a facilitator of the local diagnosis and action planning process.

iii) Group learning processes are central; Group inquiry, sharing information and interaction between outsiders (professionals) and insiders (local people).

Activities should aim at awareness raising, capacity building and empowerment of local people as well as lead to debate about change needed, action planning and implementation

iv) The major sectors in which RRA/PRA has been applied are: agriculture, livestock production and health care practices. RRA/PRA has been used to identify the needs and priorities of local people, to study specific topics and for (participatory) appraisal, planning, implementation and monitoring of development programmes. In some cases RRA/PRA has also been used to analyze gender differences in a community.

Practical Approach Towards Reaching Goals via PRA Tools

Participatory Rural Appraisal (PRA) is an exercise for communication and transfer of knowledge. Regardless of whether it is carried out as part of project identification or appraisal or as part of country economic and sector work, the learning by doing and teamwork spirit of PRA requires transparent procedures. For that reason, a series of open meetings (an initial open meeting, final meeting, and follow up meeting) generally frame the sequence of PRA activities. Other tools common in PRA are:

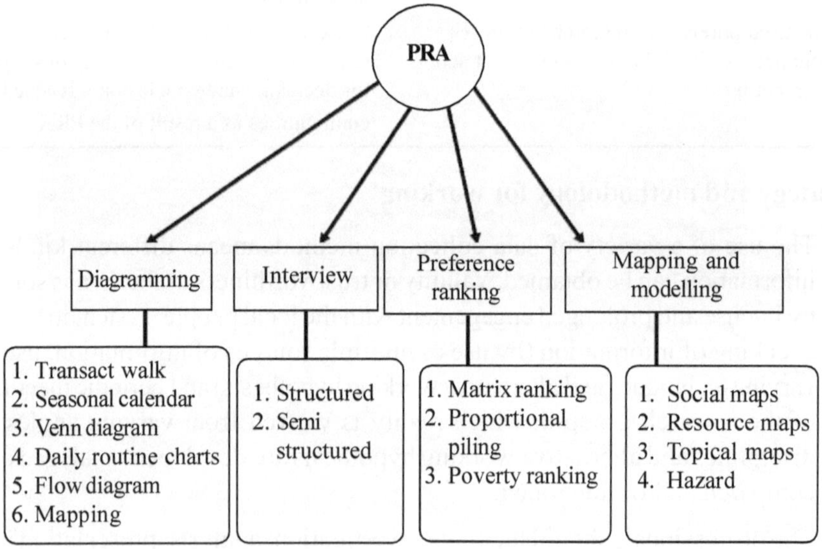

1. Diagramming

a) Transect Walk

Transects are observatory walks to study the natural resources, topography, indigenous technology, soils and vegetation, farming practices, problems and opportunities. These are done with a group of villagers-either following a particular course, cross country or covering the area.

b) Seasonal Calendar

Seasonal Diagrams can be used for obtaining seasonal patterns of rainfall, employment, income/expenditure, diseases, livestock, production, workforce availability, crop pattern etc.

c) Venn diagram

It is used to depict key institutions, organizations & individuals and their relationship with the local community or others. Key players in decision making are shown. On the Venn diagram each institution is represented by a circle. The size of the circle represents the importance, significance or power of that institutions.

d) Daily Routine Charts

It is used to identify daily routine pattern of either gender in a particular area. it helps in analyzing work type and distribution of workloads throughout the day, for comparative analysis between different individuals daily schedules. It helps:

- To identify the gender roles.
- To document the timings of the activities.
- For discussion of new activities and their implications for time use.
- For discussing time of meetings and training sessions
- To illustrate mobility and periods spent away from home.

e) Flow Diagram

Flow diagrams discover and analyze impacts and linkages. Current situations, constraints, problems and opportunities can be discussed as the effects of specific problems or interventions.

f) Mapping

Maps are used to identify the comparative location and importance of different resources with in an area. They can examine a great breadth of subject matter, and allow for a range of different types of maps to be produced for one area, or for comparative analysis by different groups with in the same area.

2. Interviewing

a) Structured

b) Semi-Structured

SSI is a tool that can be used any time. SSI is guided interviewing, where only some of the questions are predetermined and new questions come up during the interview. The interviewer prepare a list of topics and questions rather than a fixed questionnaire.

i) Individual interviews

ii) Group Interviews

iii) Key Informant Interviews

iv) Focus group discussions

3. Preference ranking

Ranking of problems, issues, solutions on the basis of needs or personal preference

a) Matrix Ranking

The main objective here is to prioritize the issues at hand such as:

It allows us to see individual and group priorities and can also be applied on the uneducated and illiterate groups in a community.

b) Proportional Piling

It is a measure of relative importance of issues and thus helps in obtaining data from respondents in relative terms. Moreover, it can also be used for questions whose answers people don't like to give directly e.g. income levels, expenditures etc.

c) Poverty Ranking

4. Mapping and Modeling

The making of maps that depicts conditions and environment of the area is called mapping. It increases the knowhow of the natives about their surrounding and the physical features of the area.

a) Social Maps

Consists of household information such as population density, social classes, land use etc.

b) Resource Maps

Shows resources of the area like soil, water, minerals etc.

c) Topical Maps

Contains information about physical features of the area, crops grown in the area, population and infrastructure facilities present in the area.

d) Hazard Maps

Showing areas that can be affected by hazards.

PRA Tool: Resource Map

Description

The Village Resource Map is a tool that helps us to learn about a community and its resource base. The primary concern is not to develop an accurate map but to get useful information about local perceptions of resources. The participants should develop the content of the map according to what is important to them.

Objectives

To learn the villagers' perception of what natural resources are found in the community and how they are used.

With whom: Female and male focus groups

Time needed: 2 hours

Key Questions

1. What resources are abundant?
2. What resources are scarce?
3. Does everyone have equal access to land?
4. Do women have access to land?
5. Do the poor have access to land?
6. Who makes decision on land allocation?
7. Where do people go to collect water?
8. Who collects water?
9. Where do people go to collect firewood?
10. Who collects firewood?
11. Where do people go graze livestock?

12. What kind of development activities do you carry out as a whole community? Where?
13. Which resource do you have the most problem with?

Social Map

Description

A social map of the kushet is a map that is drawn by the residents and which shows the social structures and institutions found in an area. It also helps us to learn about social and economic differences between the households.

Objectives

- To learn about the social structures in the Kushet and the differences among the households by ethnicity, religion and wealth.
- To learn about who is living where.
- To learn about the social institutions and the different views local people might have regarding those institutions.

Key Questions

1. What are the approximate boundaries of the kushet with regard to social interaction and social services?
2. How many households are found in the Kushet and where are they located?
3. Is the number of households growing or shrinking?
4. What are the social structures and institutions found in the Kushet?
5. What religious groups are found in the kushet? Where in the Kushet are the different religious groups living?
6. What ethnic groups are found in the kushet? Where in the Kushet are the different ethnic groups living?
7. Which are the female Headed Households and where are they are located?

Time

1,5-2 hours

Hints

- If people find it difficult to understand this tool, it will be helpful to draw a simple example for them.

- During the whole process, take care that once somebody has given a statement, you ask the others whether they agree, disagree or want to add something.
- The notetaker must ensure that all important points of the discussion and also other information is documented.
- The purpose of the social map must be very clear to all participants, make sure that the participants do not have wrong expectations. For example they might think that the poor households will get food donations, which is completely wrong.
- Unlike resource mapping, social maps need good and well prepared facilitation. Be aware that some of the issues that might be discussed could be sensitive issues for the group.
- Make sure that the objective of having all households shown on the map will be achieved.

Wealth Ranking Objectives

1. To investigate perceptions of wealth differences and inequalities in a community
2. To identify and understand local indicators and criteria of wealth and well-being
3. To map the relative position of households in a community

Methods

1. Ranking
2. Mapping

Selecting Key Informants

Carry out the exercise with a few key informants who know the community well.

Facilitator

Two PRA-team members

Key Questions

1. What are local perceptions of wealth, well-being and inequality?
2. What socio-economic groupings are there in the community and who belongs in what group?

Steps

1. A numbered list is made of all the households in the community (see social map) and the name each household head and the household number is written on a separate card.
2. A number of key informants who know the village and its inhabitants very well are asked to sort the cards in as many piles as there are wealth categories in the community, using their own criteria.
3. After sorting, ask the informants for the wealth criteria for each pile and differences between the piles. Assure the informants of confidentiality and do not discuss the ranks of individual families, so as not to cause bad feelings within the community.
4. List local criteria and indicators derived from the ranking discussion.

Example

Local Perceptions of Malnutrition Mapping Objectives:

- To identify various forms of malnutrition prevalent in the community.
- To understand the local perceptions of malnutrition.
- To map nutritionally vulnerable households

Methods

3. Key informant interview
4. Mapping
5. Ranking
6. Matrix

Selecting Key Informants

Carry out the interview with one or more key informants. Below, possible key informants are listed and ranked (1 to 4) according to priority.

1. Community Health Worker (1)
2. Traditional Birth Attendant (3)
3. Home Agent (2)
4. Traditional Healer (3)
5. Teacher (4)

Facilitator

One PRA-team member

Key Questions

3. What are the commonly seen health problems in this community? List by children, adults and women.
4. For each group (children, adults and women) can you rank these health problems according to their importance? Give ten marks to the most important problem and one mark to the last important problem. Give a mark between 1 and 10 to the remaining problems.
5. Can you explain why you have given more importance to one problem than to another? *(i.e. higher incidence, more severe, etc.)*
6. Can you identify those problems that are important for nutrition *(i.e. marasmus, kwashiorkor, night blindness, diarrhea, anemia, etc.)?*
7. For each of the nutrition-related problems, what do local people see as the causes? *(Draw a matrix with the problems, causes, treatment)*
8. What do local people in general do to treat these problems?
9. Can you identify on the village map those households that have frequently such nutrition-related problems?
10. For each of the households that you have marked, can you explain what the nutrition-related problems are?
11. For each of the households that you have marked, what are in your opinion the reasons why these households are having the nutrition-related problems that you mentioned?

Venn Diagram on Institutions

Description

The Venn Diagram on Institutions shows institutions, organisations, groups and important individuals found in the village (Kushet), as well as the villagers view of their importance in the community. Additionally the Diagram explains who participates in these groups in terms of gender and wealth. The Institutional Relationship Diagram also indicates how close the contact and cooperation between those organisations and groups is.

Objectives

- To identify external and internal organisations/groups/important persons active in the community
- To identify who participates in local organisations/institutions by gender and wealth

- To find out how the different organisations and groups relate to each other in terms of contact, co-operation, flow of information and provision of services

Key Questions

1. Which organisations/institutions/groups are working in or with the community?
2. Which institutions/groups do the villagers regard as most important, and why?
3. Which groups are addressing household food security and nutrition issues?
4. Which organisations work together?
5. Are there groups which are meant for women or men only?
6. Are some particular groups or kind of people excluded from being members of or receiving services from certain institutions?

Time

1.5 - 2 hours

Hints

If people find it difficult to understand this tool, it will be helpful to draw a simple example for them.

Seasonal Calendar

Type of group

Mixed group for women and men

Description

A seasonal calendar is a participatory tool to explore seasonal changes (e.g. gender-specific workload, diseases, income, expenditure etc.)

Objectives

- To learn about changes in livelihoods over the year and to show the seasonality of agricultural and non agricultural workload, food availability, human diseases, gender-specific income and expenditure, water, forage, credit and holidays.

Key Questions

1. What are the busiest months of the year?
2. At what time of the year is food scarce?
3. How does income vary over the year for men and women?
4. How does expenditure vary over the year for men and women?
5. How does rainfall vary over the year?
6. How does water availability for human consumption vary over the year?
7. How does livestock forage availability vary over the year?
8. How does credit availability vary over the year?
9. When are holidays and how many days in which month?
10. When are most agricultural work carried out by women?
11. When are most agricultural work carried out by men?
12. When is most non-agricultural work carried out by women?
13. When is most non-agricultural work carried out by men?
14. Which could be the most appropriate season for additional activities for men and women? What time constraints do exist and for what reason?

Time

2 hours

Hints

- Additional issues for the Seasonal Calendar may be added according to the needs and interests of the participants.

Income and Expenditure Matrix

Description

The Income and Expenditure Matrix is a tool that helps us to identify and quantify the relative importance of different sources of income and expenditures. The tool also helps us to understand how secure or how vulnerable certain groups of people incomes are. In the Expenditures matrix, we can see if all, most or only some of people's total income is spent to meet basic needs - food, water, clothing, shelter, health care, education. We can also ask whether people have any money left over to save or to invest in tools, fertilizer, or other important items that could help them in their work.

Objective

To learn about sources of income (cash and kind) and how income is proportionality spent by gender and wealth.

With whom

Two mixed focus groups (men and women), one looking at gender differences, the other at wealth differences.

Time needed

2 hours

Key questions

Income matrix

1. What are the most important sources of income in the community, both cash and in kind?
2. Who has only a few sources of income?
3. Who has many sources of income?
4. How do poor peoples sources of income compare to rich people's?
5. How do women's sources of income compare to men's?

Expenditure matrix

6. How are expenditures spread out over the year?
7. Which expenditures are common to almost every one?
8. For each social group, what proportion of income is spent on basic needs like food, clothing, housing, health care and education?
9. Who can save?
10. Who can buy equipment, tools, agricultural inputs, or other things that help improve their work?
11. How do women's expenditures compare to men's?

Hints

Discussing incomes and expenditures can be highly sensitive. People are reluctant to talk about these issues in public. Be sure to reassure the participants that you do not want to know about amounts, but will only be talking about relative proportions for each group. There will be a sensitive moment when you ask the group to agree on how to divide the stones among the rich, middle and poor groups. Be sure that you limit the total number of stones for the community as a whole. We suggest 50 stones.

Daily Activity Clocks

Description

Daily Activity Clocks illustrate all of the different kinds of activities carried out in one day. They are particularly useful for looking at relative work-loads between different groups in the community. Comparisons between clocks show who works the longest hours, who concentrates on a few activities and who does a number of tasks in a day, and who has the most leisure time and sleep.

Objectives

To learn what different people do during one day and how heavy their workloads are.

With whom

Female and male focus groups; you can also do this with focus groups of boys and girls, if there is time.

Time needed

1 hour

Key Questions

1. For each person, how is his or her time divided?
2. What is the difference between the women's and the men's clocks?
3. Who has the heaviest workload?
4. Who has time for rest and leisure?
5. How much time per day do women or girls spend collecting water and fuelwood?

Hints

You can start by drawing a picture of how you spent your day yesterday.Draw a big circle on paper and indicate when you wake up, what time you go to bed and all the activities in-between. No need to go into great detail, but be sure to show that all kinds of activities are included such as work, housework, child.

Exercise

Q.1 What is PRA and RRA? Write methodology of working for RRA.

Q.2 Plan and execute awareness programme for livestock farmers regarding health care practices with the help of RRA/PRA.

14

Planning and Organization of Group Discussion

Group Discussion

Group discussion is the method by which two or more persons meet, express or suggest their ideas for getting the solution to the felt problems by them.

Objectives of group Discussion

- To develop the democratic leadership among the members.
- To conduct the systematic group discussion to solve the problems.
- To give opportunity to each member to share experiences.
- To promote the habit of talking, thinking, group planning and group action.
- To identify the group and focus the public interest and mobilize them for group action.

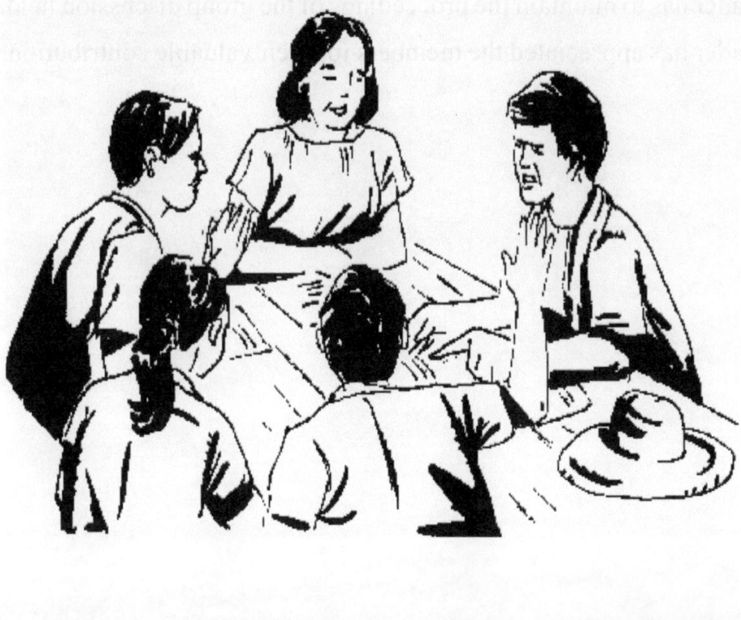

Procedure to conduct group discussion

1. Invitation for minimum 20 to 25 people for informal group discussion.
2. The date, time and venue of meeting is decided and communicated to the people in advance.
3. The seating arrangement of group discussion should be in circular or semicircular fashion.
4. The group members decide the group leader democratically.
5. At the start of the meeting of the group the leader welcomes members.
6. The problem or the topic is communicated to members to discuss and to get solution at the end of the discussion.
7. As being a member of the group each and everybody has to share his experiences with respect the subject or problem.
8. If anybody is not sharing himself during the discussion then group leader has to take lead and discuss the problem at his level.
9. If any member is discussing the problem continuously for long time or other than the subject then group leader has to inform him that he had given nice ideas, next one please.
10. During the group discussion the group leader has to write the important points of each spokesman with his name.
11. At the end the group leader has to read the problem with solution and the action plan suggested by the members of the group.
12. Group leader has to maintain the proceedings of the group discussion held.
13. Group leader has appreciated the members for their valuable contribution.

15

Self Help Groups - An Overview

Introduction

India with exceeding population of 1027.01 million with 741 million living in rural areas is on the path of development. The lack of access to and control over resources is said to be cause of poverty (Satapathy and Mishra, 2011).

Women form half of our society. They have significant role in overall development. Rural development concept in our country attaches more importance to women empowerment. To combat poverty 'self help promotion' is of recent paradigm that has attracted attention to sections of the society.

Self Help Group (SHG)

A self help group (SHG) is a village-based financial intermediary usually composed of 10–20 local women or men (Ramchandran, 1995). Members make small regular savings contributions over a few months until there is enough capital in the group to begin lending. Funds may then be lent back to the members or to others in the village for any purpose. In India, many SHGs are 'linked' to banks for the delivery of microcredit.

It can be defined as a homogenous group of rural people, voluntary governed to save whatever the amount they can conveniently save out of their earnings and mutually to contribute to a common fund to lend to the members for making their production and emergency consumption credit needs (Patil and Patil, 2012).

History of SHGs

The SHG concept is not new to India. The traditional Indian society functioned mainly on the basis of self- help and mutual- help. A common bond like caste, sub-caste, blood kinship and the place of congenial atmosphere links the members. The Seva Gram concept of Gandhiji also stressed on this.

SHGs have emerged as a means of providing poor people with the credit that they need to emerge from poverty. The Grameen Bank was started in 1976 by

Professor Mohammed Yunus in response to this need for capital by the poor. Later in 1983 it was converted into a statutory body by an ordinance of the government of Bangladesh. The Grameen Bank disbursed loans to groups consisting of five women; six to eight groups formed a centre (Misra, 2011). The Grameen Bank used group guarantees, developed compulsory savings mobilization among the groups of poor people and had decentralized, cost effective operations for lending to the poor (Mc Guire and Conroy, 2000).

Groups were formed in MYRADA in 1984-85 and were initially called credit management groups. In fact several Non Government Organizations (NGO's) notably Professional Assistance for Development Action (PRADAN) working in Rajasthan and Tamil Nadu realized that the Integrated Rural Development Programme (IRDP) system of provision for credit to the poor was ruining the banks as well as the poor. They experimented with lending to groups and persuaded banks to lend to such groups.

A review by the working group on bank lending to the poor through NGOs and SHGs led to policy changes that enabled banks to lend to groups, which were not formally registered, and without knowing the purpose of advance (Mahajan and Ramola, 2003, Fernandez 2007). In Tamil Nadu, the government supported programme began in 1989 as an IFAD assisted pilot project in two blocks in Dharmapuri district, through the women's development corporation of Tamil Nadu (Gariyali and Vettivel, 2003).

SHGs were also set up in Andhra Pradesh in 1992. It started as a total literacy campaign in Nellore district which led to the anti arrack movement. At a village meeting in Leguntapadu, the district magistrate suggested the savings of a rupee a day by women, leading to the formation of savings and credit groups. (Ramchandran, 1995). In Maharashtra NGOs like Chaitanya and Bharatiya Agro Industries Foundation (BAIF) have been active in forming SHGs for over fifteen years.

Objectives of SHGs (Gurumoorthy, 2000)

1. Basically the SHGs are economic organization. Small funds are raised for day to day needs. The saving groups when transformed to earning groups not only increase the productivity of women but the credibility also.
2. SHGs improve life style and living standard of members.
3. As economical solutions are available, the family structure is maintained.
4. SHG is a good way to stop the exploitation of consumers.
5. Total rural economy is improved by increasing family income of individuals.

6. Broadening of view is a major gain. The ascending order of family, group, village, Tehsil, Zilla, Zone, State, Nation, World, makes the vision global.
7. Development of self-confidence is achieved.
8. A common platform is available for a dialogue and sharing of views.

Growth of SHG in India

The SHG bank linkage project is expected to be advantageous to the banking sector from both the angles of fulfilment of social goals (like reaching out the poor) and achieving operational efficiency (by externalizing part of their transaction cost). The improvement of the SHG bank linkage programme is seen in Table 3. In the initial period i.e. in 2000-01, just 263825 SHGs were linked to banks with Rs.4808.70 million as refinance from NABARD (Shinde and Ingole, 2011). In a span of one and half decade it is expanded rapidly. In 2006-07 20, 2924973 SHGs have been linked with the banks with refinancing of Rs.1, 80,407 million.

So as far as spatial outreach of the SHG bank linkage is concerned the programme covered 583 districts in 31 states/UTs. The state wise SHG bank linkage data shows that the programme is skewed in favour of the southern states, particularly Andhra Pradesh. This state alone accounts for 26.2 per cent of total SHGs formed and 38.1 per cent of the total credit, while the North-East and Northern region together constitutes 8.7 per cent of the total programme. This imbalance is an issue that requires serious attention. It needs sustained effort in other regions where there is a latent demand for microfinance services.

Table 3: Growth of SHG in India

Year	Cumulative No. of Groups	Cumulative amount of loan (Rs. in millions)
2000-01	263825	4808.70
2001-02	461478	10260.00
2002-03	717360	20490.00
2003-04	1079091	39040.00
2004-05	1618456	68984.60
2005-06	2238565	139754.30
2006-07	2924973	180407.40

(Shinde and Ingole, 2011)

How to Start a SHG? (NABARD, 2005)

Even a thousand-mile journey starts with a single step forward.

The first step for forming a SHG is also simple

- Visit the very poor families in concerned village.
- It is important to be known to the people and to win their trust.
- Talk to the elders in the village, explain your plan to them and request for their support.
- Speak to the women folk.
- Ask what the most important issue for the family is?
- Every time when you visit such families, it should be cleared that you are not distributing or promising any subsidy money under any scheme. This is very
- This is called 'Preliminary Survey'. This helps you to understand the needs of each individual family.
- When you see them for the second time, you will be able to tell each family how you have seen and spoken to other families, who also have very similar
- By visiting the families, you will be able to know which of those families could come together in self-help groups.

Stages in Group Development (Puhazhendi and Satyasai, 2001)

Earlier studies have suggested that groups move through stages but these are not constant across different groups. Groups are shown to be in four stages:

Group formation - 0-6 months

Group stabilization - 7-12 months

Self reliance - 13-18 months

Institutionalization - 19-24 months

Misra (2003) categorizes these stages as

1. **Formation:** Where the formation revolves around the solution of a common problem. The discordant members should not become part of the same group, as it leads to waste of time and energy in resolving the disputes.
2. **Stormative:** When the group struggles to cohere some members who cannot co-exist with others may have to leave. Thus, the first few months will see this transition.
3. **Normative:** After the group settle down, it will decide on issues relating to transaction of business such as how much to save, when a bank account should be opened, who should keep a record of the meeting, etc.

4. **Performative:** This is gained once the loan cycle has been completed and the NGO and SHG both gain stability. The group expands its programs.

Training of the group members is carried out in a number of subjects; they are taken on exposure visits, disseminated information and are constantly monitored as regards their development (Tankha, 2002).

How are group meetings organised? (Harpar, 2002)

- This is called community participation.
- This is the right time to tell everyone that the meetings are not for "giving" anything, but to "enable" the poor families to come together and help each other.
- It will be very useful if you explain the basic principles of SHG in this meeting.

How do SHGs take shape?

- After meeting the elders and community leaders, you are now ready to call SHG members for a meeting. This can be called "a start up meeting".
- Please allow sufficient time for the members to understand the different aspects of group formation.

Membership

During the initial meetings, following things may happen-

- Some members leave.
- Some new members come.
- They want to remain together and help each other.

Leadership (Shetty, 2002)

One member of the group needs to take the lead. To identify the person following questions should be ask within the group:

Questions	Answers
Who should decide everything for the SHG?	All members should decide
Who benefits from the SHG?	All members benefit
Who should do the work?	All should share the work
How can the work be shared?	Agree on one person to take up the work by rotation

This way, the members will understand the reason for rotation of the responsibilities. This will make it easy to choose a member to take initiative for the following main activities:

- Book keeping
- Organising meetings

How do SHGS Function? (Yadav, 2003)

Simple rules are required for SHGs to function. The following are some important rules:

- Common agreement on when to meet
- Agreed penalties for non-attendance
- Agreement on amount of saving
- Giving small loans to each other
- Taking loan from banks, repayment habits

Training of the members is an important need for proper functioning of SHGs

Trainings can be provided in the following areas:

- Basic mathematics
- Writing of books
- Basics of lending money, borrowing and repaying

Book Keeping by the SHGs

- Simple and clear books for all transactions to be maintained.
- If no member is able to maintain the books, someone to be engaged by the group for the purpose.
- Animator can also help. (Parikh, *et al.*, 2006)

1. **Minutes Book** The proceedings of meetings, the rules of the group, names of the members, etc. are recorded in this book.
2. **Savings and Loan Register** Shows the savings of members separately and of the group as a whole. Details of individual loans, repayments, interest collected, balance, etc. are entered here.
3. **Weekly Register** Summary of receipts and payments on a weekly basis which should be updated on every meeting.

4. **Members' Passbooks** Individual members' passbooks encourage regular savings.

Activities of SHGs (Sheik Mohemed, 2004)

- Loans to members
- Community action
- Common investment
- Increase employment, income and saving
- Better living

Functions of SHGs

a) Savings and Thrift

- The amount may be small, but savings have to be a regular and continuous habit with all the members.
- 'Savings first -Credit later' should be the motto of every group member (Singh, 2005).

b) Internal lending

- The savings to be used as loans for members.
- The purpose, amount, rate of interest, etc., to be decided by the group itself.
- Proper accounts to be kept by the SHG.

c) Discussing problems

- Every meeting, the group will discuss and try to find solutions to the problems faced by the members of the group.

Linking of SHGS to Bank (NABARD, 2004)

STEP 1: Opening of Savings Bank Account for the SHGs

- The Reserve Bank of India has issued instructions to all commercial banks and regional rural banks, permitting them to open SB A/c of registered or unregistered SHGs.
- SB A/c in the name of SHG could be opened after obtaining the following documents from the group.

Resolution from the SHG

The SHG has to pass a resolution in the group meeting, signed by all members, indicating their decision to open SB A/c with the bank. This resolution should be filed with the bank.

Authorisation from the SHG

The SHG should authorise at least three members, any two of whom, to jointly operate upon their account. The resolution along with the filled in application form duly introduced by the promoter may be filed with the bank branch.

A savings bank account passbook may be issued to the SHG. This should be in the name of the SHG and not in the name of any individual/s.

STEP 2: Conduct of Internal Lending by the SHGs

- After saving for a minimum period of 2 to 3 months, the common savings fund should be used by the SHG for lending to its own members.
- The purpose, terms and conditions for lending to its members, rate of interest etc., may be decided by the group through discussions during its meeting (RBI and NABARD have permitted the members to decide on these aspects). Simple and clear books of account of savings and lending should be kept by the SHG.

STEP 3: Assessment of SHGs

- We need to know whether the SHG has been functioning well or not. The check list given below will help us to assess each SHG in a simple, but effective manner.

Table 4: Check list to assess the performance of a SHG

S. No	Factors to be checked	Very good	Good	Unsatisfactory
1.	Group size	15-20	10-15	Less than 10
2.	Type of members	Only very poor members	2 or 3 not very poor	Many not poor members
3.	Number of meetings	4 meetings in a month	2 meetings in a month	Less than 2 meetings in a month
4.	Participation of members	Very high level of participation	Medium level of participation	Low level of participation
5.	Savings collection within the group	4 times a month	3 times a month	Less than 3 times a month
6.	Amount to be saved	Fixed amount	Varying amount	-
7.	Utilization of savings amount by SHG	Fully used in loaning to members	Partly used for loaning	No proper utilization
8.	Loan recoveries	More than 90%	70-90%	Less than 70%
9.	Maintenance of books	All books regularly maintained and updated	Only some are maintained	Irregular in maintaining
10.	Accumulated savings	More than Rs. 5000/-	Rs. 3000-5000/-	Less than Rs. 5000/-
11.	Educational level	More than 20% of members can read and write	-	Less than 20% of members can read and write

(NABARD, 2005)

STEP 4: Sanction of Credit Facility to the SHGs

In whose name is the loan issued?

The loan is always sanctioned and issued on the name of SHG. (Not in the name of the individual members).

What is the quantum of loan? How is the quantum decided?

The amount of loan to the SHG can be to the tune of 1 to 4 times of its savings.

What constitutes the savings of the group?

- The group's balance in the savings bank A/c
- Amount internally lent amongst the members
- Amount received as interest on the loans

What are the purposes for which the loan can be given to the SHG?

The purpose can be emergency needs like illness in the family, marriage, etc. or buying of assets for income generation acquisition of assets. The group will discuss and decide about the purpose for which loans are to be given to its individual members by the SHG (Yadav, 2003).

Who makes the repayment?

The SHG makes the repayment to the bank (group is collectively responsible for the repayment of the loan).

What is the collateral security for the bank?

RBI/NABARD rules stipulate that no collateral security should be taken from SHGs by banks.

Collateral security is not necessary for the loans sanctioned to SHGs because:

- The members of SHGs know that the bank loan is their own money like savings.
- They are aware that they are jointly responsible for the repayment.
- Therefore, they exert moral pressure on the borrowing members for repayment.
- Because of this, the bank gets a much better repayment from the SHG.

What is the rate of interest to be charged for the loans granted to SHG by the bank?

The Reserve Bank of India has allowed the banks freedom to decide on the interest rates to be charged to the SHGs.

What is the rate of interest to be charged by the SHGs to its members?

The rate of interest to be charged by the group to its members should be left to the group. This is usually 2 or 3 rupees per hundred rupees of loans.

List of documents required by banks for lending to SHGs (Singh, 2005)

i) Inter-se agreement to be executed by all the members of the SHG
ii) Application to be submitted by SHG to bank branch while applying for loan assistance (This includes details of the purposes for which the SHG gives loan to its members).
iii) Articles of agreement for use by the bank while financing SHGs.

It is generally seen that in most of the SHGs, the maximum number of members are married, are age group of 30-40 years, and having some education. There is an increase in monthly income of family approximately Rs. 4000-6000. (Patil and Patil, 2012).

Empowerment activities-Different empowerment activities of SHGs in agriculture and allied sectors

Table 6: Empowerment activities of SHGs

S.No	Major Areas	Specific Areas
1.	Agriculture	Seed production
		Rice processing
2.	Horticulture	Raising seeds Vegetable cultivation
		Floriculture
		Vermicompost
		Mushroomcultivation
		Bee keeping
3.	Fishery	Fingerling production
4.	Livestock	Poultry rearing
		Goat/Sheep rearing
		Dairy Piggery
5.	Bi-products	Bamboo workLeaf plate making

(Satapathy and Mishra, 2011)

Empowerment of Women Through Animal Husbandry SHGs

Besides agriculture, women are involved in most of the operations in animal husbandry enterprises like dairy, poultry, rabbit rearing and mushroom cultivation. Women participated in activities having economic significance like cattle management, poultry keeping, sheep rearing, preparing manure and carrying manure. In animal husbandry women have a multiple role. Their activities vary widely ranging from care of animals, fodder collection, cleaning of animal sheds to processing milk and livestock products.

In livestock management indoor jobs like milking, feeding, cleaning etc are done by women in 90 per cent of families, but more than 90 per cent of rural women in India are unskilled in livestock rearing lead them to earn low income. Still most of them carried out in traditional rearing pattern face loss in the enterprise. If they train in scientific livestock rearing practices by new technology interventions mainly in feeding certainly help them to earn more profit. When the technologies properly introduced and adopted by the respondents it will improve the production and reproduction status of the animals. The change in the income pattern will be assessed (Reddy, 2007). The waste from livestock will be converted into organic manure like vermin compost and panchagavya.

Major Components of the Empowerment (Vidya, 2006)

1. Establishing scientific livestock rearing units through changed feeding pattern by green fodder, azolla and agro-by-products etc.
2. Feeding, breeding and disease control will be given due care by introducing suitable technologies.
3. Value addition of milk and meat produced from the animals.
4. Preparation of vermin compost and panchagavya.
5. Construction of biogas plant wherever possible and slurry management.
6. Promotion of organic farming.
7. Assessing the change evolved by introducing technology and increased income.

Measures of Empowerment

Women throughout the world have been subject to gender discrimination in varying forms. They also remain under-represented in decision –making and hold less than 10 per cent of seats in parliament in most region of the world (King and Mason, 2001)

They are subject to laws that discriminate against them violence at home and outside and are under represented in parliament and legislature (Kumar and Sen, 2003).

Women, especially among the poor work longer than men in unpaid household level activity, this restricts their participation, income generation and decision making. Hence, these needs have to be raised cautiously after first meeting (Vidya 2006). Some of the strategic needs of women that need to be addressed are:

- Reduced vulnerability to violence
- More economic security
- More options and opportunities
- Shared responsibilities with men for reproductive work
- Increased ability to improve the lives of their children

- Networking with other women for solidarity
- Increased political power

Hence programmes aimed at empowering women must measure the interventions which have in fact enhanced women's space in decision making, whether, it had increased their access to credit, finances, property, nutrition, education, health care and whether it has decreased violence against women and whether it has improved their status in society and participation in governance.

Social Impact and Empowerment (Shinde and Ingole, 2011)

Women comprised a majority of the SHG members. The impact on empowerment was measured on various parameters of self-confidence seen from self-worth and communication skills, Behavioural changes seen from desire to protest against social evils, response to problem situations and family violence.

Self confidence

Members' feelings of self-worth as assessed by looking at their confidence level, treatment received from family members, attitude in helping the neighbours. While 20 per cent of the pre group members displayed confidence, 88 per cent of post SHG group members exuded confidence. 63 per cent of the post SHG group members experienced better treatment by family members.

Communication skills

While 88 per cent of members did not talk freely during the pre group period, 77 per cent expressed that they could talk freely in the post group period. 72 SHGs from Orissa, Uttar Pradesh, Maharashtra and Karnakata has also registered improvement in the diet, assets and education of the members, though the benefits to the poorer members was found to be more delayed.

- **Influence on her own development:** The decisions considered were whether she had the freedom to choose her own income generating activity and whether she could join in adult learning programmes or add to her educational status.
- **Power over local polity:** The issues looked at were, the involvement of the member in group formation, SHG meetings, involvement in political activities like elections, commercial activities like involvement with banks, promoter NGOs, meetings at panchayat level-projection of her views at these meetings, parliamentary, state and village elections.

- **Improvement in technical and managerial skill:** Skills learnt to undertake on farm or off farm income generation activities, to moderate a meetings successfully, to resolve conflicts among SHG members.

Mobility

91.9 per cent of new group members reported having gone to the nearest town, and 85.9 per cent old group members and 85.5 per cent new group members reported having gone to a city. Thus, the level of mobility was quite high.

Financial Position

89 per cent of members from old groups reported a positive influence on their share in the family income as compared to 71 per cent of members from new groups. Thus the improvement in economic status by being part of the SHG is undisputed. 74.2 per cent of old group members reported an increase in the share in family income as against 50 per cent of new group members.

Confidence level

More of the members of older groups reported an increase in confidence levels in dealing with individuals and institutions than the members in new groups.

Knowledge about health and hygiene

Awareness about child's vaccination, using toilets at home and adding fruits and vegetables to the diet of a pregnant women was greater among the members of older groups than among the new groups (Jain, 2003).

Ownership of house and land

Also 32 per cent of members of older groups reported owning residential land and 18 percent owned farmland as compared to 17 per cent of new grip members who owned residential land & 12.9 per cent who owned farmland. This point to the positive effect of being part of the SHG enhancing women's property rights.

Change in role in decisions about self

65 per cent of members in older groups reported that the control over their own lives had improved as compared to 48.4 per cent of members of new groups.

Participation in local affairs

40 per cent of members from old groups participate regularly in the Gram Sabha as compared to 17.7 per cent of members from newer groups.

Decisions affecting the family

Regarding schooling of the girl child, 31.3 per cent of members from the old groups decided on their own as compared to 16.1 per cent of members from new groups, joint decision with husband was 32.8 per cent and 33.9 per cent respectively (Agrawal, 2001).

The study thus concludes that the members of the old groups emerge as more confident, financially more secure, more in control of their lives. Hence we can conclude that the process of empowerment seems to have started in the old groups.

Weakness of SHGs (Satapathy and Mishra, 2011)

- Group conflict
- Caste and class dominancy
- Unequal benefit sharing
- Market fluctuation
- Lack of formal rules and regulations
- Male interference
- Weak account and record keeping
- Lack of group inter-relationship
- Lack of credit accessibility
- Lack of market cooperatives

Conclusions

- The evidence of women's empowerment through SHGs provides a varied picture. The women empowerment is in a better position to negotiate the use of the loans taken by them to take up gainful activity and participate in the marketing of their products.
- However, there is a need for a more in-depth analysis of the SHGs in India in order to ascertain whether the increase in women's access to credit has had similar negative impacts in increasing their susceptibility to violence within the family.
- The overall multi-faceted development for women by SEWA can be contrasted with the now harsh reports remerging about the Grameen Bank, especially in its recovery style. The difference seems to be that SEWA is an organization run by women, for women, while the Grameen Bank seems to

have emerged as an organization run by men through loans in women's names.

- Rather women, who have bettered themselves a little, prefer to withdraw to the sell of home based activity, leaving the 'outside' world to be transacted by men, without violating the traditionally held norms of women being part of the private space within the household, rather than part of the public space outside it.
- The importance of the process of group formation and the development of groups ethos in building sustainable SHGs clearly seem to emerge as a necessary factor for the success of SHGs. However, it is not only the provision of credit which leads to the empowerment of the members of the groups, but the sustained inputs in conscentisation of the women and raising their level of awareness by means of sustained capacity building.
- The SHGs act as a support group developing courage and offering mutual solace and comfort to the members. It is when training in accounts and managerial inputs are given, that the availability of credit leads to the setting up of successful ventures. This success in turn leads to a growth of their confidence and improves their status at home and in the community.

References

Agrawal, D., (2001). Empowerment of rural women in India. Social Welfare, 48(4): 3-4.

Deshmukh, R.J., (2004). Women's participation in self help groups and in Panchayati Raj Institutions: suggesting synergistic linkages. Ind. J. For Gender Studies, 5(2): 5-7.

Fernandez, P., (2007). Knowledge for development effectiveness, History and spread of self help group affinity movement in India. International Fund for Agricultural Development. Agricultural Development and Practical Action Publishing Ltd. Pp. 24-56.

Gariyali, C.K. and S.K.Vettivel, (2003). Women's own: The self help movement of Tamilnadu. Self Help Group. Vetri publishers. Pp.9.

Gurumoorthy, T.R, (2000). Self Help Groups Empower Rural Women. Kurukshetra, 3(5) Pp.31-37.

Harpar, M.,(2002). Promotion of self Help Groups under the SHG Bank Linkage Programme, NABARD, New Delhi. Indus Publishing Company. Pp.22-24.

Jain, R., (2003). Socio-Economic Impact through Self Help Groups. Yojana, 47(7):11-12.

Kant, S.K., (2001). Woman's Empowerment and Mutual Cooperation in the Family. Social Welfare, 48(1):3-4.

King and Mason, (2001). Women economic empowerment as the "Magic Potion" of development. Women economic empowermen. Bain & Company publishers. Pp 5-6.

Kulkarni, V., (2006). The Self Help Group Movement- Women in Local Governance, Ind. UNICEF, 12(1)4-7.

Kumar, A. and B. Sen (2003). Health inequity and women self help group in India: The role of caste and class. Health Sociology Rev., 16(5):160-168.

Mahajan, V. and B. Ramola (2003). Microfinance performance of public sector banks in the NER of India. J. of appl. mang. and computer sci., 4: 57-80.

Mc Guire, P.B. and J.D.Conroy (2000). Getting in framework right: Policy and regulation for microfinance in Asia, Foundation for development cooperation. Wilson's publications. 5(2): 234-300.

Misra, R.K. (2011). Women empowerment through self help group in India. Ind. Streams Res. J., 1(2):44-55.

Mishra, S.J.(2003). Self help group development in India. Pp.3-5. http://www.ifad.org/evaluation/public_html/eksyst/doc/.../india-13.htm

NABARD. (2004). Reports, Progress of SHG bank linkages in India, 2003-2004: 60-79.

NABARD. (2005). Annual Report,. Progress of SHG bank linkages in India, 2001-2002: 15-17.

Parikh, Tapan. S.,K. Sasikumar., and S. Olanganathan, (2006). Promotion of quality book keeping in Self Help Group, The small enterprise education and promotion network. Thompson Press. Pp.2-4.

Patil, S.J. and Y.S.Patil, (2012). Role of self help group (bachatgat) in development of rural economy. Asian J. of Res. in Business Economics and Manag., 2(8):92-105

Persai, S., (2010). Women Empowerment Project Tejaswini in MP. Pp.2-3. http://www.orchha.org/Selfhelp.php.

Puhazhendi, V. and Satyasai, K.J.S., 2001: Economic and social empowerment of rural poor through SHGs. Ind. J. of Agric. Economics, 56(3):56-63.

Ramchandran, R., (1995). Organizing self help group with disabilities. Asia and Pacific J. on Disability., 2: 223-41.

Reddy, C.S., (2005). Self Help Group- A Keystone of Microfinance in India. Pp. 11-12. http:// www.empowerpoor.org.htm

Reddy, K.R., (2007). Women Empowerment. SHG Federations in India. Enable Publishers. Pp. 45-50.

Satapathy, C., and Sabita Mishra., (2011). Formation and activity of Self Help Group. SHGs in Techno Economic Empowerment of Tribal Women. New India Publishing Agency. Pp. 11-117.

Sheik Mohamed, (2004). Self help group for the success of Women Entrepreneurs. Kissan World, 52(8): 41-43.

Shetty, S.L.,(2002). Working and Impact of Rural Self help Groups and other forms of Microfinancing. Ind. J. of Agric. Economics, 57(1): 31-32.

Shinde, K.H., and Prof. Ingole P.S., (2011). Women Empowerment through Self Help Group in India. Ind. Streams Res. J., 1(4): 3-5.

Singh, A.K,. (2005). SHG bank linkage model-wise cumulative position upto 31st March, 2005. NABARD. 20-39.

Tankha , A., (2002). A study prepared for ICCO and Cordaid. The Netherlands, 3(4): 15.

Thapa, G., (2011). Sustainability and Governance of Microfinance Institutions: Recent Experiences and Some Lessons from Southeast Asia. Asian J. of Agric. and Development, 3(1):23-25.

Yadav, V.K., (2003). Reports, Progress of SHG bank linkages in India, 2002-2003 NABARD. Pp.7-20.

16

Educational Technologies for Effective Extension Services in Rural India

1. Introduction

"Educational Technology is the application of scientific knowledge about learning and the conditions of learning to improve the effectiveness of teaching and training. In the absence of scientifically established principles, educational technology implements techniques of empirical testing to improve learning situation".

Educational technology includes numerous types of media that deliver text, audio, images, animation, streaming video that includes technology applications and processes such as computer-based learning as well as local intranet/ extranet and web-based learning. Information and communication systems whether free-standing or based on either local networks or the internet in network learning underlie many e-learning processes (Tavangarian *et al.*, 2004).

The role of Educational technology is to develop veterinary research, education and extension to improve quality of life in rural area. Educational technology can help an average Indian farmer to get relevant information regarding livestock and agriculture inputs, crop production technologies, food processing, market support, livestock finance and management of farm business. The extension mechanism is becoming dependent on educational technology to provide appropriate and location specific technologies for the farmers to furnish timely and proficient advice to the farmers.

Educational technology can be a best mean not only to develop extension but also to expand research and education system.

2. Concept of Educational Technology

Educational technology is the effective use of technological tools in learning. As a concept, it concerns an array of tools such as media, machines and networking hardware as well as considering underlying theoretical perspectives for their effective application.

2.1 Association for Educational Communications and Technology (AECT)

AECT denoted educational technology as "the theory and practice of design, development, utilization, management, and evaluation of processes and resources for learning" (Lowenthal and Wilson, 2010).

2.2 National centre for programmed learning, UK

"Educational technology is a complex, integrated process involving people, procedures, devices and organization for analyzing problems and devising implementing, evaluating and managing solutions of those problems involved in all aspects of learning" (Lucido and Borado, 1997).

2.3 Richey

Richey defined educational technology as "the study and ethical practice of facilitating learning and improving performance by creating, using and managing appropriate technological processes and resources" (*Richey, 2008).*

3. History of Educational Technology

Abacus

The invention of the abacus in 3,000 BC marked the beginning of computers. For the first time, people had a calculating device.

Saun-Pan and Soroban

The earliest surviving counting board is the Salamis Tablet which dates back to 400 BC. China (Saun-pan) and Japan (Soroban) introduced computer trays at about the same point in history (200 AD). The Soroban (a type of abacus) is still used today for calculating.

Stonehenge

Around 2,300 BC the creators of Stonehenge first began work on what is now known as an astronomical calculator. This miraculous complex took over 2,000 years to complete. Stonehenge stands on Salisbury Plain, two miles west of the town of Amesbury, Wiltshire, in Southern England.

Leonardo da Vinci Calculator

In 1452 AD it is believed that Leonardo da Vinci conceived of a calculation device.

Guttenburg Printing Press

Johannes Gutenberg (Germany) developed the printing press, sometimes considered the greatest invention of all time. Between 1452 and 1456, Gutenberg printed the first book ever, the Bible.

Napier's Bones

John Napier, the inventor of logarithms, created an aid to calculation known as 'Napier's Bones' in 1617. He described a method of multiplication using "numbering rods" with numbers marked off on them. Napier's numbering rods were made of ivory, so that they looked like bones. This explains why they are now known as Napier's bones. To multiply numbers, the bones were placed side by side and the appropriate products read off.

Slide Rule

Robert Bissaker first created the slide rule in 1654, an instrument used by engineers and scientists until the 1970s. The slide rule was a precursor to the electronic calculator.

Magin Cataoprica

The Magin Catacoprica or magic lantern, invented in 1646, led to the eventual zoetrope. Magic lantern, or slide, shows played an important role, attracting young and old to schools, theaters, and homes to watch depictions of fables, legends, and current events. The magic lanterns projected hand-painted or photographic glass slides, which were inserted into the projector one at a time for small audiences to view together. A skilled projectionist could move them quickly, making the screen images appear to move.

Jacquard Loom

In 1725, Joseph-Marie Jacquard (French) invented a way to weave silk using punched cards. These punched cards would become the predecessors of those used in the first computers. The idea of using punched cards to control machines was considered to be the birth of modern day computer programming.

Benjamin Franklin-Electricity

Benjamin Franklin discovered electricity when he flew his kite one stormy day in June, 1752. This discovery would eventually allow us to power the computers we have come to rely on so heavily in our modern society.

Charles Babbage's calculating engines

Charles Babbage's calculating engines (1822) are among the most celebrated icons in the prehistory of computing. Babbage is often considered the "Grandfather of Modern Digital Computing". He was the first person to realize that a computing machine must be composed of:

- Input device (the card reader)
- Memory (the store),
- Central processing unit (the mill),
- Output device (the printer).

Telephone

In1876, Alexander Graham Bell invented the electrical speech machine is a telecommunications device that permits two or more users to conduct a conversation when they are too far apart to be heard directly. A telephone converts sound, typically and most efficiently the human voice, into electronic signals suitable for transmission via cables or other transmission media over long distances, and replays such signals simultaneously in audible form to its user (Annabel, 2002).

Kinetoscope

In the late 1800s Thomas Edison invented the Kinetoscope, The Kinetoscope is an early motion picture exhibition device. The Kinetoscope was designed for films to be viewed by one individual at a time through a peephole viewer window at the top of the device.

Wireless Communication: Radio

In 1894 the young Italian inventor Guglielmo Marconi began working on the idea of building a commercial wireless telegraphy system based on the use of Hertzian waves (radio waves), he successfully sent signals between a transmitter and a receiving antenna. Marconi's apparatus is also credited for saving the 700 people that survived the tragic Titanic disaster (Sungook, 2001).

Educational Film

The earliest forerunners of the educational film were the scientific motion picture. In 1902 Charles Urban exhibited films which showed the growth of plants, emergence of a butterfly, & undersea views. These films are thought to be the first educational films. Thomas Edison was one of the first to produce films for classrooms.

Television

The first public demonstration on television was conducted in 1927. Television or TV is a telecommunication medium used for transmitting moving images in monochrome (black-and-white) or in color and in two or three dimensions and sound. It can refer to a television set, a television program or the medium of television transmission. Television is a mass medium for entertainment, education, news, and advertising (Helmis and Jacob, 2003).

Differential Analyzer

Bush Vannevar, an American scientist from 1919 to 1971 Bush worked and taught at Massachusetts Institute of Technology (MIT) where he invented the differential analyzer, a forerunner to the modern computer.

Turing Machine

Turing, a British Mathematician, often known as the founder of computer science, developed the Turing machine in 1936. Turing's Machine is the cornerstone of the modern theory of computation and computability even though it was invented nine years before the creation of the first electronic digital computer.

Old filmstrip projector

Filmstrip projectors were a simpler alternative to slide projectors. Filmstrips were used from the 1940s to the 1980s. Teachers would load a roll of film with static images into the projector. Many filmstrips came with a phonograph record (later a cassette tape) with the narration. An audible beep would indicate when to move to the next image. Some film strips simply came with a script for the teacher to read, while later model projectors could auto-advance based on sub-audible tones embedded in the cassette tape.

Mini-Computers

Mini-computers and BASIC were both introduced in 1964. A minicomputer, or mini, is a class of smaller computers that developed in the mid-1960s. A machine costing less than US$25,000, with an input-output device such as a tele printer and at least four thousand words of memory, that is capable of running programs in a higher level language, such as Fortran or BASIC. Minis were designed for control, instrumentation, human interaction, and communication switching as distinct from calculation and record keeping (William and Smith, 1970).

Pocket Calculator

During 1972, three engineers from Texas Instruments, Kilby, Maryman and Van Tasel, invented the electronic pocket calculator.

Smart board

The Smart Board is a line of interactive whiteboards produced by david Martin and Nancy Knowlton in 1991 through their company Smart Technologies. The Smart Board interactive whiteboard operates as part of a system that includes the interactive whiteboard, a computer, a projector and white boarding software either Smart Notebook collaborative learning software for education, or Smart Meeting Pro software for business. The components are connected wirelessly or via USB or serial cables. A projector connected to the computer displays the desktop image on the interactive whiteboard. The whiteboard accepts touch input from a finger, pen or other solid object. Smart Board interactive whiteboards are also available as a front-projection flat-panel display interactive surfaces that fit over plasma or LCD display panels (Dvorak, 2012).

Mobile Phone

Mobile phone is a portable telephone that can make and receive calls over a radio frequency carrier while the user is moving within a telephone service area. The radio frequency link establishes a connection to the switching systems of a mobile phone operator which provides access to the public switched telephone network (PSTN). Most modern mobile telephone services use a cellular network architecture and therefore mobile telephones are often also called cellular telephones or cell phones. In addition to telephony 2000s era mobile phones support a variety of other services such as text messaging, MMS, email, Internet access, short-range wireless communications, business applications, gaming, and digital photography. Mobile phones which offer these and more general computing capabilities are referred to as smart phones. The first handheld mobile cell phone was demonstrated by Motorola in 1973 (Kelmens, 2010).

4. Scope of Educational Technology

Educational technology refers to the use of both physical hardware and educational theoretic. It encompasses several domains, including learning theory, computer-based training and online learning where mobile technologies are used such as m-learning. Accordingly, there are several discrete aspects to describe the intellectual and technical development of educational technology:

- Educational technology as the theory and practice of educational approaches to learning
- Educational technology as technological tools and media that assist in the communication of knowledge, and its development and exchange
- Educational technology for learning management systems (LMS), such as tools for student and curriculum management, and education management information systems.
- Educational technology itself as an educational subject; such courses may be called "Computer Studies" or "Information and Communication Technology" (ICT).

5. Objectives of Educational Technology

'Make instructions more powerful learning more immediate and access more equal' (Venkataish, 1995). Objective is often classified as general and specific.

5.1 General Objectives

- Organizing effective educational systems, behaviors, methodologies, communication, learning environment and education evolution.
- Creating, inventing, developing, researching, evaluating and circulating educational technology and communication innovations that are appropriate for instructor in various groups of subjects.
- Educational technology explores emerging technical possibilities in the context of education.

5.2 Specific Objectives

- To bring fullest, all round development of individual in terms of physical, mental, moral and social development.
- To develop in man, ability to think and take sound decisions to solve the problem (Rathakrishnan *et al.*, 2009).

6. Purpose of Educational Technology

- The purpose of education technology is "to make education more productive and more individual, to give instruction a more scientific base and to make instruction more powerful, learning more immediate and access more equal (Tickton, 1971).
- Educational technology prescribes the design of instruction material, structures learning interaction for maximum benefit.

- Education technology is an effort with or without machines to manipulate the environment of individuals for generating a change in behavior of learning (Knezevich and Eye, 1970).

7. Need of Educational Technology

- Educational technology can make an ordinary person capable of superior performance and a means either printed or electronic to distribute that instruction.
- Educational technology provides ways and means of integrating hardware and software teaching aids (Rathakrishnan *et al.*, 2009).

8. Importance of Educational Technology

- Educational technology aids to improve the process of human learning "Educational technology is a complex integrated process involving people, procedures, ideas, devising, implementing, evaluating and managing solutions to those problems involved in all aspects of human learning"
- Educational technology connects processes and products of instructional design.
- Educational technology aims at improving all aspects of communication i.e., encoding, message, channel, barrier, decoding, retention and application.
- Educational technology deals with the process of implementing methods and resources with regard to group dynamics and individual diffusion.
- Educational technology based on psychology and social anthropology, it is a system with the number of interconnected and interdependent components.
- Educational technology principles are applicable to all topics and subjects hence basic to all communication development (Rathakrishnan *et al.*, 2009)

9. Types of Education Systems

Three types of education systems are:

9.1 Incidental

9.2 Non-formal

9.3 Formal

9.1 Incidental Education/ Informal education

Incidental education is all that one learns as a concomitant of growing up in the society. It is the life long process by which every person acquires and accumulates knowledge, skill, attitudes and insights from daily experiences and exposure to the environment at home, at work, at play etc. (Coombs and Ahmed, 1974).

9.2 Non-Formal Education.

It is a organized systemic educational activity carried on outside the framework of the formal system to provide selected type of learning to particular groups in the population adults as well as children according to their needs. Example, Agricultural Extension (Coombs and Ahmed, 1974)

A. Methods of Non-formal Education

Non-formal education is based upon techniques of communication other then classroom interaction. One can reach out by correspondence through audio visual resources as the learners can conveniently use. Depending upon the means of communication and the state of art in education technology different modes of non-formal education are as follows:

a) Correspondence Education b) Distance education

c) Open Learning/open programme d) Continuing education Programme

a) Correspondence Education

In most Universities, correspondence education courses run separately from the regular formal education. Students are separately enrolled and offered courses through print-matter posted to them. Correspondence courses run by some professional tutorial companies to prepare the students for competitive admission examination have become very popular. Students may, therefore, continue their school studies in the forenoons and take up correspondence courses for the self study in the afternoon and evening at their convenience. Correspondence courses are liked by the adult learners who do not like or cannot attend the fixed time courses. They do not come to know about others attending the same courses; no one knows whether they are taking the course or lagging behind others, except if there are short-term personal contact programmes.

Correspondence courses may be offered through the media of audio and video cassettes or through other means of communication. However, financial restraints usually limit them to print-matter.

b) Distance education

Distance education is like formal education except that a physical distance separates the teacher and the student, teachers employ all the techniques of correspondence education with personalized tutorials by using mass media, i.e., radio, news-sheets and television.

Distance education aims at making the education available at the doorstep of the learner. It takes the education to remote places rather than require the learners to come from remote places to any fixed place of learning such as reversal of formal education has found a place in society where a very large number of learners are scattered all over the country, some parts of which may be physically inaccessible. With the ongoing population explosion and people living below the poverty line, distance education provides a ray of hope.

c) Open Learning/open programme

Open learning experiments were initiated in the UK in early sixties. Success stories resulted in the establishment of the premier Open University at Milton Keynes in the UK. They have since introduced degree and diploma courses in almost all subjects in arts, sciences and engineering. Their researches have led them to believe that high quality print-matter together with audio-visual resources is the most effective when combined with arranged tutorials. After this in India the Indira Gandhi National Open University (IGNOU) was established in September 1985 with its head quarters in South Delhi.

Open universities employ all possible techniques and technologies to educate their students. They have access to radio, television broadcasts and they have their own infrastructure to produce all types of audio and video programmes. They employ the mode of distance education as the methods of study -circles, group tutorials, tutored video instruction, etc by hiring space and faculty, wherever necessary open learning is the most flexible of all.

d) Continuing education programmes

It refers to the learning of working professionals at any time during their career. They may take short or long courses in institutions. Alternatively, live university lectures are transmitted for reception by all those enrolled for the course. If that is not possible, video cassettes of recorded lectures are dispatched by courier service to them immediately after the lectures. Advances in educational technology are thus employed in educating the working professionals without disrupting their normal routine.

9.3 Formal Education

Formal education is highly institutionalized, chronologically graded and hierarchically structured education system spanning lower primary school and the upper reaches to the university (Coombs and Ahmed, 1974)

The formal systems of education came from eighteenth century. The formal elementary schools were highly useful. The modern system of formal education has been created and has grown to tremendous dimensions as elementary, primary, secondary and higher secondary education (Rathakrishnan *et al.*, 2009).

10. Educational Technology Initiatives for Effective Extension Services In India

a) Kissan Mobile Sandesh, Madhya Pradesh

In 1983 the KVK Chindwara has started KMS service aiding instant bulk messaging from KVK to individual farmers, extension personnel and agro input providers for extending agricultural information through bulk SMS. Five development blocks from Chindwara and Seoni district were selected for study. This service has found extremely cost effective with strong storage facility for rural farmers. KMS is being used as a medium to send information on important training and other programmes to contact farmers of KVK (Wankhade *et al.*, 2010).

b) Akshaya-Malappuram, Kerala

The Akshaya project, first started in the rural Malappuram district of Kerala in 2002, was the first district wide e-literacy project in India and one of the largest known Internet Protocol (IP) based wireless networks in the world. A joint project between local bodies (gram panchayats) in rural areas, municipalities in urban areas and private entrepreneurs in Malapuram district of Kerala was started to bridge the digital divide by providing community access to internet and computers with a goal at least one person in every family to be computer literate in that district. About 2662 Akshaya e-centres are in rural areas. The project offers lots of services like: E-Pay, E-Krishi (for farmers to provide online agriculture trading and information portal, E-Vidya, E-Ticketing, online medical transcription course and village kiosk for all extension programs.

c) Self employed women's association (SEWA)-Ahemdabad, Gujrat

SEWA is a large primary trade union that has about 1.9 million registered women working since 1972 in the informal sector. These are women who earn a living through their own labour or small businesses. They do not obtain regular salaried employment with welfare benefits like workers in the organized sector. SEWA started using the Sat Com (satellite communication) programme in 1998 with its receiving terminals in nine districts and transmitting terminals in Gandhinagar. SEWA's two main goals are full employment and self reliance SEWA has started computer training, marketing facilities, vocational training for semi-literate women workers. Many of its milk cooperatives are using computerized milk collection software.

d) AMUL milk collection system-Anand, Gujrat

The Anand Milk Union Limited (AMUL) was established in 1956 before the promulgation of the Gujarat State Cooperative Act, 1961. AMUL with more than 578,000 members was the first cooperative dairy to be established in Anand, Gujrat. AMUL introduced an automatic milk collection system in 691 milk collection centers which reduced the time required for collecting the milk. The system weighs the milk and measures its fat content at time of delivery to the centre and this has enabled immediate payment to the farmer.

e) The Dairy Information and Services Kiosk(DISK), Gujrat

It is one of the successful initiatives taken up by Gujarat Cooperative Milk Marketing Federation Ltd (GCMFL) with the help of Indian Institute of management, Ahmedabad. DISK aimed at helping the dairy farmers with timely messages and educating them on the care for their milch cattle and enhance the production of quality milk. It also aims at assisting the dairy unions in effectively scheduling and organizing the veterinary, artificial insemination, cattle feed and other related services.

It is being used at milk collection centers and in cooperatives to measure butter fat content of milk test the quality of the milk and promptly make the payment to the farmers. It has resulted in the removal of incentives to those who adulterate milk, reduced the time for payments from 10 days to less than 5 minutes and instilled the confidence in farmers on cooperative set up (Haque, 2000).

f) Community information centers (CICs)-Gangtok, Sikkim

The Community Information Centre (well known as CIC) Project has been implemented on pilot basis in 30 blocks of the North Eastern states & Sikkim in India This project was started by the department of information technology, Government of India with the technical support of the national informatics centre (NIC) on 17th August 2002. Presently, all 4876 blocks in 79 districts of the 8 states, basic services to be provided by CICs include Internet Access, E-mail, Printing, Data entry & Training for the local people. In addition e-Suvidha, Prices & other market information of Agricultural & Veterinary produce (Chamling, 2015).

f) n-Logue Chiraag Kiosks, Chennai

Chennai based India's largest operator of for profit rural kiosks under "Chiraag" brand, established in 2005-06, focusing on fee based transactional services.

Chiraag kiosk provides a substantial number of informational services using content that is localized and stored on site include education and training, healthcare, agriculture consultancy and e-governance (Jhunjhunwala *et al.*, 2004).

g) Janmitra-Jalawar, Rajasthan

This project is a joint initiative of United Nations Development Programme and the Government of India operational since 2002. It has been implemented with the help of district administration Jalawar, Department of information technology and Rajcomp, a state agency. It provides e-governance, e-education, e-health and e-commerce services to the villagers through 30 community information centers (CICs); 21 departments are connected to the server through dial up connectivity and 13 departmental offices are on local area network (LAN) with the server.

i) Village Knowledge Centers (VKCs),Pondicherry

Village knowledge centers of MS Swaminathan research foundation were launched in 1998 in Pondicherry. The main aim behind the establishment of VKCs was to provide sustainable food security in rural areas of Pondicherry. To fulfill this aim, it provides technical information related to agricultural inputs. It helps in procuring quality seeds, in providing information about the daily marked priced from the government as well as private bodies, and advices farmers on rotation of crops as well as about the use of fertilizers and pesticides. VKCs receive information by voice mail, and disseminate it through any public address system. It has also identified 13 districts in Pondicherry, where there is a huge potential for agriculture business, and where the government will invest Rs. 170 crores (Saravanan *et.al*, 2011).

j) HP I Community in Kuppam

HP launched the world's first i-community or inclusive-community at Kuppam in February 2002. Three years later, the citizens of Kuppam, around 300,000 in number, have access to Information & Communication Technology based solutions to everyday life situations - solutions that also have long ranging social and economic benefits, as well, thereby helping this rural region grow faster. Informational services of Kuppam are offering information on government programs and contacts, agriculture and veterinary information, information on employment, education and health. Self help group management information and computer training are also offered.

11. Some of the Important Efforts by Public Sector, NGOS and Private Sector in Educational Technology for Rural Development in India (Vivek, 2011)

- Cyber extension program of MANAGE (http://www.manage.gov.in/)
- National Informatics Centre (NIC) (http://home.nic.in)
- Community Information Centre (CIC) (http://www.cic.nic.in/)
- e-Seva (http://www.esevaonline.com)
- N-Logue (http://www.n-logue.co.in/home.htm)

12. SWOT Analysis (Strengths, Weakneses, Opportunities and Threats) of Educational Technology in India

12.1 Strengths

- On farm solution of the problems
- Facilitation of internet at the doorstep of the farmers
- Transfer of technology becomes faster
- Improved farm productivity and standards of living in rural community
- Improve market access to farmers

12.2 Weakness

- Lack of awareness among users
- Lack of realistic financial model
- The projects have not adequately transferred capabilities to rural areas
- Lack of facility for training farmers in regional languages
- Lack of financial support by the government
- Lack of effective communication and coordination

12.3 Opportunities

- Work area can be expended to neighboring villages and states
- Employment generation in agriculture and allied sectors

12.4 Threats

- Frequent strikes
- Shortage of electricity lead to deterioration of project
- Initial cost is high which cannot afforded by the farmers

13. Conclusion

The Indian farmer and those who are working for their welfare need to be e-powered to face the emerging scenario of complete or partial deregulation and reduction in government protection, opening up of agricultural markets, fluctuations in agricultural environment and to exploit possible opportunities for exports. The quality of rural life can also be improved by quality information inputs which provide better decision making abilities. Educational technology can play a major role in facilitating the process of transformation of rural India to meet these challenges and to remove the fast growing digital divides.

The rapid change in the field of educational technology makes it possible to develop and disseminate required electronic services to rural India. The existing bottlenecks in undertaking the tasks need to be addressed immediately. A national strategy needs to be drawn for spearheading educational technology penetration to rural India. A national coordinating agency with an advisory role can act as a catalyst in the process.

No single institution or organization alone can succeed in the task of e-powering farmers and rural India. At the same time scattered and half hearted attempts cannot be successful in meeting the objective. Industries with major stake in villages should come together to provide the initial impetus.

The success of any educational technology based service to rural India hinges on evolving a proper revenue model for the dissemination points. The information kiosks can draw revenue from the industry by providing and disseminating required services. Once these dissemination points prove to be economically viable, the educational technology revolution in rural India will require no crusaders (Mittal, 2012).

References

Annabel, Z.D. (2002). The Essential Guide to Telecommunications. Prentice Hall PTR, New Jersey, 183p.

Coombs, P.H and Ahmed, M. (1974). Attaking Rural Poverty: How Non Formal Education Will Help. The John Hopkins University Press, Baltimore. 8p.

Chamling, P. (2015). Sikkim Exploring the Newer Frontiers, 2nd Edn., Surya Printographics, New Delhi, pp 338-354.

Dvorak, R. (2012). SMART Board Interactive Whiteboard. John Wiley & Sons, London, Pp 12-23.

Haque, S.M. (2000). The diminishing publicness of public service under the current mode of governance. Public administration review, Hyderabad. 1(61): 65-82.

Helmes, M. and Jacobs, J. (2003). The Television History Book. British Film Institute, Queensland, pp 11-54.

Jhunjhunwala, A. Ramachandran, A. and Bandyopadhyay, A. (2004). n-Logue: The Story of a Rural Service Provider in India. The Journal of Community Informatics, 1(1): 30-38.

Knezevich, S.G and Eye, G.G (1970). Instructional Technology: Past, Present & Future, 2nd Edn., American school Of School Administrators, Washington DC, 16p.

Kelmens, G. (2010). The Cellphone: The History and Technology of the Gadget That Changed the World. MacFarland & Company, North Carolina, pp 45-53.

Lucido, P.I. and Borabo, M.L. (1997). Educational Technology, Katha Publishing Co., Quezon City, 5p.

Lowenthal, P.R. and Wilson, B.G. (2010). Labels do matter! A critique of AECT's redefinition of the field. TechTrends, 54(1):38–46.

Mittal, S.C. (2012). The Role And Potential Of Information Technology In Agricultural Improvement. Economics of Agriculture, 61:471-485.

Richey, R.C. (2008). Reflections on the 2008 AECT Definitions of the Field. TechTrends, 52 (1): 24–25.

Rathakrishnan, T., Isreal T.M. and Nirmala, L. (2009). Advances and Challenges in Agricultural Extension and Rural Development, New Delhi Publishing Agency, New Delhi, pp 22-31.

Sungook, H. (2001). Wireless: From Marconi's Black-box to the Audion, MIT Press, Cambridge. pp 20-22.

Sarawanan, R., Kathiresan, C. and IndraDevi, T. (2011). Information and Communication Technology for Agriculture and Rural Development, New India Publishing Agency, New Delhi, pp 50-55.

Tickton, S.G. (1971). To improve learning: An evolution of instructional technology, R.R Bowker Company, New York, 32p.

Tavangarian, D., Leypold, M., Nölting, K. and Röser, M. (2004). Is e-learning the Solution for Individual Learning?. Journal of e-learning, 2(2): 273–280.

Venkataish, V. (1995). Implementing Computer Technologies: Teachers' Perceptions and Practices, Journal of Technology and Teacher Education, 14(1): 173-207.

Wankhade, A., Khare, N., Pannase, S. and Shrivastava, D. (2010). ICT based Kisan Mobile Sandesh – An Innovation Approach. In:Sarawanan, R., Kathiresan, C. and Indra Devi, T. (ed.). Information and Communication Technology for Agriculture and Rural Development, New India Publishing Agency, New Delhi, pp.143-146.

Vivek, A. (2011). Cyber Extension: A Convergence of ICT and Agricultural Development. Global Media Journal, 2(2):1-8.

William, D. and Smith. (1970). Maxi Computers Face Mini Conflict: Mini Trend Reaching Computers. New York Times, 3p.

17

Practical Tools for Gender Analysis

Women account for 43% of the agricultural labor force in developing countries (FAO, 2011) and produce 50% of the global food production (FAO, 2011). Regional statistics reveal that in Latin America about, 20 percent, in Asia, about 30 to 60 percent, and in Sub-Saharan Africa, 50 to 75 percent of the agricultural labour force is supplied by women (FAO, 2013). Moreover, they invest 10 times more than their male counterpart in the family well being especially education and nutrition of children (Maertens and Verhofstadt, 2013). Despite being the primary contributors for the world food production, their roles are highly underestimated. Considerable gender bias exists in the agricultural sector, both in terms of quantities of assets, agricultural inputs and resources that women control (Deere *et al.,* 2013). Failure to recognize the roles, differences and inequities [between men and women] poses a serious threat to the effectiveness of the agricultural development agenda (World Bank, 2009). Gender inequalities and lack of attention to gender in agricultural development contribute to lower productivity, lost income, and higher levels of poverty as well as under nutrition (Peterman *et al*., 2010).

An increase in women's capacity to manage different aspects of a given system will enhance the capacity of that system to innovate and sustain itself. Gender-responsive agricultural policies have contributed to overcoming asymmetries in gender power relations, especially where they provided structures and mechanisms for improving women's access to assets including information, training, land, and technology (World Bank, 2009). But for making robust policies especially for the empowerment of women the developers need solid information regarding the real conditions of the people. Usually socio economic analyses provide this specific information to policy makers (U.N.D.P., 2001). But the general routine analyses of the socio economic conditions fail to analyse the specific problems of women, since the dimensions of gender inequalities are deeply embedded making it difficult to perceive, hence it requires a more specialized frameworks. The varied strategic and practical needs of women compared to men compelled the policy makers and social scientist to develop novel techniques to analyse their socio-economic needs.

Gender analysis is a sub-set of socio-economic analysis (UNDP, 2001). These analyses disclose how gender relations affect a developmental programme. Its aim is to highlight the fact that gender relations are likely to impact on the solution of problem and it also indicate what is the impact likely to be and the alternate course of action (Ochola, 2010). Since the societies throughout the world is permeated by gender differences and gender inequalities (U.N.D.P., 2001), implementation of any programme which is gender neutral can in fact reflect or probably exacerbate that difference. Gender analysis can be said as a process that helps to collect, identify, examine and describe the roles and activities of men and women and also highlights the key factors contributing to inequalities between them (Ludgate, 2016). It explores and highlights the relationships of women and men in society, and the inequalities in those relationships, by asking: Who does what? Who has what? Who decides? How? Who gains? Who loses? (March *et al.,* 1999). It also asks which men or women did the task. (*ibid*). Gender analysis breaks down the divide between the private sphere (involving personal relationships) and the public sphere (which deals with relationships in wider society). It looks at how power relations within the household interrelate with those at the international, state, market, and community level. In short, gender analysis represents the variety of tools and approaches that can be used to understand the relationship between men and women, their access to and control over resources, and their constraints and opportunities they face relative to each other (Ludgate, 2016). The primary aim of gender analysis is gender equity rather than gender equality.

Gender analysis and Extension

In the present decade, one of the key objectives of extension is gender mainstreaming. Since these analyses systematically gather and examine the information on gender differences and social relations, in order to identify, understand and re address the inequalities based on gender, it is a valuable diagnostic tool for extension policy makers and workers.

It help to access the participation of men and women in extension activities and how to tailor the programme as per their needs. Understanding the different role and responsibilities also help the extension workers to make specific agricultural programmes that increases income and yields as well as alleviate the drudgery of both the gender (ibid). According to Ludgate (2016), the gender analysis helps the extension agents to:

- Distinguish the roles of men and women in agriculture, their enterprises and tasks, resources and use of end-products.

- Identify the root causes of existing gender disparities and propose strategies to address them (e.g., access to information).
- Identify different needs and priorities of men and women in both the near- and long-term.
- Examine traditional power imbalance between men and women and identify ways to address it.
- Find ways to enhance women's participation and share of benefits from extension interventions.
- Find ways to provide information to men and women as it relates to their specific tasks, responsibilities, interests and needs.

Conducting a gender analysis

Several frameworks and methodologies are available to conduct gender analysis in development related field. The choice will depend on task in hand, the context and the resource available (March *et al.,* 1999). Some framework (eg :Harvard Framework) gives more importance to micro planning and gender roles whereas others emphasis enquiry into social relations and others have been exclusively designed to look at women empowerment. Since the frameworks select a limited number of factors from a huge number of factors affecting the situation, it reflects only a crude face of reality. In the context of extension each situation and programmes are different. So the selection a framework for a particular programme depends on the interplay of values and assumptions of developers of programme. The extension agent can use a particular framework or combine two or more frameworks or modify a particular framework by adding innovative ideas, as per his or her need. Whatever is the approach, bare minimum information is required to conduct a gender analysis in agriculture is given below:

1. Ideas about women's and men's role
2. Factors that shape gender and Gender division of labour
3. Access and control over resources and their distribution system
4. Analysis practical and strategic needs and interest of men and women
5. Assessing the barriers and constraints faced by men and women.

Since there is no framework which suits all the context or situation, prior experience of the extension worker / planer in that context, will aid in identifying the most suitable framework. In case of novice extension personals, before selecting a particular framework, it would be ideal to have a formal discussion with experienced counterparts, followed by an analysis of strengths and limitation of each framework.

Common tools used in Gender analysis

1. Harvard Analytical Framework

The Harvard Analytical Framework is also called the Gender Roles Framework or Gender Analysis Framework. Developed by the Harvard Institute for International development in collaboration with the WID Office of USAID, and based on the WID efficiency approach, it is one of the earliest gender analysis and planning frameworks.

Aims of the Harvard Framework

- To demonstrate that there is an economic rationale for investing in women as well as men.
- To assist planners in designing more efficient projects and improve overall productivity.
- To emphasize the importance of better information as the basis for meeting the efficiency/equity goal.
- To map the work of men and women in the community and highlight the key differences.

Features

The framework consists of a matrix for collecting data at the micro- (community and household) level. It has four inter-related components:

1. The activity profile, which answers the question "who does what?", including gender, age, time spent and location of the activity.
2. The access and control profile, which identifies the resources used to carry out the work identified in the activity profile, and access to and control over their use, by gender.
3. The analysis of influencing factors, which charts factors that influence gender differences in the above two profiles;
4. The project cycle analysis, which examines a project or intervention in light of gender-disaggregated information.

The framework also contains a series of checklists consisting of key questions to ask at each stage of the project cycle: identification, design, implementation and evaluation.

Uses

- Best suited for project planning, rather than program or policy planning;
- As a gender-neutral entry point when raising gender issues with constituents resistant to considering gender relations and power dynamics;
- For baseline data collection;
- The gender frameworks rely on the economic argument of most efficient allocation of resources. It therefore uses language similar to that of economists, which can be particularly useful when talking to people whose main influence is mainstream economic thought.

Strengths

1. Its practical and hands on
2. Give a clear picture of gender division of labour
3. Distinguish between access and control of resources
4. Easily adaptable
5. Non threatening and gender neutral, rely on facts rather than theory
6. Once the data have been collected, it gives a clear picture of who does what, when and with what resources. It makes women's roles and work visible.

Limitations

1. The framework is highly focused on efficiency rather than equity
2. Tend to be over simplifying, because of superficial "tick the box" approach. Planners can end up feeling over-confident, assuming that they know all they need to know. They can thereby miss the complexities of the community's reality, and can miss crucial opportunities for change.
3. It is basically a top-down planning tool, excluding women's and men's own analysis of their situation.
4. Do not address the culture and context of the institutions which determine the allocation of resources to recipients
5. It does not delineate power relations or decision-making processes. Therefore, the framework offers little guidance on how to change existing gender inequalities.
6. Emphasizes separation of activities and resources based on sex or age, ignoring connections and cooperative relations across these categories. This can result in projects that may have unintended consequences or cannot tackle women's strategic gender needs.

2. The Moser framework

This framework was developed as part of Gender and Development approach, which argued for an integrated gender-planning perspective in all development work, concentrating on the power relations between women and men (March *et al*., 1999). Caroline Moser developed it as a method of gender analysis at the Development Planning Unit (DPU), University of London, UK in the early 1980s. Moving from analysis into action, Caroline Moser, with Caren Levy of the DPU, further developed it into a gender policy and planning method. It is based on the concepts of gender roles and gender needs, and policy approaches to gender and development planning.

Aims of Moser Framework

Moser Framework aims to set up 'gender planning' as a type of planning in its own right: 'The goal of gender planning is the emancipation of women from their subordination, and their achievement of equality, equity, and empowerment. This will vary widely in different contexts, depending on the extent to which women as a category are subordinated in status to men as a category. The Moser Framework questions assumptions that planning is a purely technical task. Moser characterises gender planning as distinct from traditional planning methods in several critical ways: firstly gender planning is both political and technical in nature. Second, it assumes conflict in the planning process. Third, it involves transformatory processes. Fourth, it characterises planning as "debate".

Features

The Moser Framework contain three concepts.

- Women's triple role;
- Practical and strategic gender needs
- WID/GAD policy approaches /policy matrix

Women's triple Role

This tool includes making visible the gender division of labour. It can be carried out by mapping all the activities of men and women (can include girls and boys) in the household over a twenty four hour period. A triple role for low income women is identified by Moser productive, reproductive and community management roles.

Productive work: This is work that produces goods and services for consumption by the household or for income and is performed by both men and women. Women's productive work is often carried out alongside their domestic and childcare responsibilities (reproductive work) and tends to be less visible and less valued than men's productive work.

Reproductive work: This work involves the bearing and rearing of children and all the tasks associated with domestic work and the maintenance of all household members. These tasks include cooking, washing clothes, cleaning, collecting water and fuel, caring for the sick and elderly. Women and girls are mainly responsible for this work which is usually unpaid.

Community roles: Women's community activities include provisioning and maintenance of resources which are used by everyone, such as water, healthcare, education. These activities are undertaken as an extension of their reproductive role and are normally unpaid and carried out in their free time. In contrast it is mainly men who are involved in politics at the community level. This work may be paid or unpaid but can increase men's status in the community.

Practical and strategic gender needs

Women have particular needs because of their triple role as well as their subordinate position to men in society. Women's needs differ from men's needs. A distinction is made between practical gender needs and strategic gender interests/needs

Practical gender needs: Women and men can easily identify these needs as they often relate to living conditions. Women may identify safe water, food, health care, cash income, as immediate interests/needs that they must meet. Meeting women's practical gender needs is essential in order to improve living conditions, but in itself it will not change the prevailing disadvantaged (subordinate) position of women. It may in fact reinforce the gender division of labour.

Strategic gender interests/needs: Strategic gender interests/needs are those that women themselves identify as due to their subordinate position to men in their society. They relate to issues of power and control, and to exploitation under the sexual division of labour.

WID/GAD Policy Matrix

The WID /GAD policy matrix provides a framework for identifying/evaluating the approaches that have been (or can) be used to address the triple role, and the practical and strategic gender needs of women in programmes and projects.

Five different policy approaches viz., Welfare, equity, anti poverty, efficiency and empowerment have been used in these evaluations.

Uses

- For planning at all levels from policies to projects;
- In conjunction with Harvard framework
- Training for awareness-raising, programme planning, and implementation

Strengths

- Accessible and easily applicable
- Moves 'planning' beyond technical concerns
- Speaks to planners in their own 'language
- Challenges inequality
- Powerful tools of practical and strategic gender needs
- The concept of the triple role makes all areas of work visible
- Distinguishes between policy approaches and thus encourages questioning an intervention's purpose.

Limitations

- The idea of gender roles obscures the notion of gender relationships and can give the false impression of natural order and equality;
- The framework does not mention other forms of inequality, such as class, race or ethnicity.
- The framework is static and does not examine change over time as a variable;
- The policy approaches should not be seen as mutually exclusive; they may often overlap each other in practice.

3. Gender Analysis Matrix

The Gender Analysis Matrix (GAM) was developed by Rani Parker, in collaboration with development practitioners working for a Middle Eastern NGO. The main theme of this matrix is participatory planning. GAM is flexible enough to handle situation where data analysis is severely handicapped. i.e. it can accommodate the constraints imposed by shortage of funding and time, illiteracy, and insufficient or non-existent quantitative data on gender roles.

Aims

GAM aims to help determine the different impact development interventions have on women and men, by providing a community-based technique for identifying and analysing gender differences. The GAM is a transformatory tool, in that its use is intended to initiate a process of analysis by community members themselves. It encourages the community to identify and constructively challenge their assumptions about gender roles.

Features

GAM is based on 3 Principles

1. All requisite knowledge for gender analysis exists among the people whose lives are the subject of the analysis.
2. Gender analysis does not require the technical expertise of those outsidethe community, except as facilitators.
3. Gender analysis cannot promote transformation unless it is carried out by the people being analysed.

The GAM features two main concepts on a matrix which focuses on the impact of a development intervention.

The GAM worksheet

	Labour	Time	Resources	Culture
Women				
Men				
Household				
Community				

The GAM analyses the impact of development interventions at four levels of society viz: women, men, households, and community. They appear on vertical level of matrix. It also analyse the impact at four areas viz labour, time, resources (access and Control) and socio cultural factors. They appear at horizontal level of matrix.

Uses

- A participatory planning tool
- It has high potential for raising awareness of women's subordination as a result of unequal gender relations. So useful for transformatory gender training.

Strength

- Designed specifically for community-based development workers
- Simple and systematic; uses familiar categories and concepts
- Transformatory as well as technical
- Fosters 'bottom-up' analysis through community participation
- Considers gender relations between women and men, as well as examining what each category experiences separately
- Levels of analysis can be added to in order to suit particular interventions
- Can be used to capture changes over time
- Helps anticipate resistance, and encourages consideration of what support should be offered for those at risk
- Can be used for participatory impact assessment
- Quick data collection

Limitations

- Needs a good facilitator
- Some factors can get lost because categories have many aspects
- Requires careful repetition in order to consider change over time
- Does not seek out the most vulnerable community members
- Excludes macro- and institutional analysis
- Difficulties defining a community
- Risk of misleading outcomes due to power relations between funders and community members.

4. Women Empowerment framework

This framework was developed by Sara Hlupekile, a gender expert from Lusaka, Zambia.

Aim

To achieve women's empowerment by enabling women to achieve equal control over the factors of production and participate equally in the development process.

Features

The framework argues that poverty arises not from lack of productivity, but from oppression and exploitation. It conceptualizes five progressive levels of equality, arranged in hierarchical order, with each higher level denoting a higher level of empowerment. These five levels of equity are:

1. Control: Using the participation of women in the decision-making process to achieve balance of control between men and women over the factors of production, without one in a position of dominance.
2. Participation: Pertains to women's equal participation in the decision-making process, policy-making, planning and administration.
3. Conscientization: pertains to understanding the difference between the sex roles and gender roles and the belief that gender relations and gender division of labour must be fair and agreeable to both sides and not based on domination of one over another
4. Access: Pertains to women's access to factors of production of three-fourths land, labor, credit, training, marketing facilities, and all publicly available services and benefits three-fourths on an equal basis with men. Equality of access is obtained by securing equality of opportunity through legal reform to remove discriminatory provisions.
5. Welfare: Pertains to level of material welfare of women, relative to men, with respect to food supply, income and medical care, without reference to whether women are themselves the active creators and producers of their material needs.

The framework also distinguishes between women's issues (equity with men) and women's concern (traditional and subordinate, sex stereotyped gender roles).

Uses

- Particularly useful for groups committed to promoting equality and empowerment through their work.

Strengths

- Develops the notion of practical and strategic gender needs into a progressive hierarchy.
- Shows that empowerment is an essential element of development and enables assessment of interventions along this criterion.
- Has a strong political perspective, aims to change attitudes.

Limitations

- Assumptions of levels of equality as strictly hierarchical is questionable.
- Framework is static and takes no account on how situation changes with time.

- Examines gender relations from the point of equity alone.
- Ignores other form of inequality.

Conclusion

The frameworks discussed above are practical instruments, designed to help their users integrate a gender analysis into social research and planning. They are a few other frameworks which are not cited here, they too can be employed if needed. When deciding which framework to use for any particular situation, it is important to consider what aspects are appropriate in your work, and what purpose you are trying to achieve because each framework was developed for a particular context. The conceptual difference between each framework must be thoroughly comprehended before selecting one. Finally, it is essential to remember that no framework will do the work for you. It may help you plan the work that can be done to confront women's subordination. But the work must be still done.

References

F.A.O. (2011).Women in agriculture: Closing the gender gap for development. The state of food and agriculture, FAO, Rome, Italy.

Maertens, M. and Verhofstadt, E. (2013). Horticultural exports, female wage employment and primary school enrolment: Theory and evidence from Senegal. Food Policy, 43: 118-131.

Deere, C.D., Oduro, A.D., Swaminathan, H. and Doss, C. (2013). Property rights and the gender distribution of wealth in Ecuador, Ghana and India. J. Econ. Inequality, 11(2): 249-265.

World Bank (2009). Gender and agriculture: Sourcebook, World Bank, Food and Agriculture Organization, and International Fund for Agricultural Development, Washington, D.C.

Peterman, A., Behrman, J. and Quisumbing, A. (2010). A Review of Empirical Evidence on Gender Differences in Nonland Agricultural Inputs, Technology, and Services in Developing Countries. IFPRI Discussion Paper 00975, International Food Policy Research Institute, Washington, D.C.

Ochola, W. O., Sanginga, P.C. and Bekalo, I. (2010). Managing Natural Resources for Development in Africa.

U.N.D.P. (2001). Gender and Development programme, UNDP learning Pack-gender mainstreaming, New York.

Ludgate, N. (2016). What is gender analysis?- Intergarting Gender and nutrition within Agricultural Extension Services, Feed the Future, Florida. Accessed from: www.agrilinks.org

March, C., Smyth, I. and Mukhopadhy, M. (1999). A guide to Gender-analysis framework, Oxfam Publications, New York.